Revie

Dr. Chaney has an engaging and … ing scientifically inaccurate information with meticulously documented research. His listing of the popular diets with the pros and cons of each is of immediate practical use. This book is a keeper!

Nedra Sahr, C.N.S., nutritionist and author of
The Fresh Start Cleansing Program

I've spent the last 11 years working with over 36,000 health and fitness experts around the world in 96 countries. I know the best of the best. And Dr. Chaney is world class expert when it comes to leading scientific research on health and nutrition today. He personally 'walks the walk' and knows the challenges each of us go through in connecting scientific research to the real world when it comes to the foods we eat. His passion on nutritional health shines through in his writing and commitment to share his knowledge and wisdom with others.

"Slaying the Food Myths" is a fantastic book for anyone looking for just the right balance of cutting edge scientific research with practical day-to-day advice for those committed to optimal health. Keep this book in your home and share it with your loved ones. It will not only assist you in solving health challenges, but you'll find answers to common questions the traditional news media seems to get wrong each week when it comes to nutrition, supplementation, and our health. If you're confused by the myths and hype out there… look no further than this book to lay out the facts and truth for living optimal health.

Sean Greeley, CEO, NPE, 8 times Inc 500/5000
Global Fitness Business Coaching Company

With his new book, in a concise and entertaining way, but with rigorously documented research, Dr Chaney guides the reader through the labyrinth of myths and maze of spurious research pertaining to the field of nutrition. This book is the perfect companion for anyone looking for answers and healthy choices regarding their daily food consumption.

Dr. Pierre-Yves Dubois, DC, Trained as a
Chiropractic Physician in Switzerland;
America's Top Chiropractor in 2009;
Advisory Board Member of Health
Network Solutions NC in 2012.

Once again, our favorite professor is cutting through the confusion and setting the record straight ... with science no less! He walks us through what the "studies" really show ... and help save us from falling prey to clever marketing ads and articles.

Barbara Lagoni, BS in Food Science and Nutrition,
Cornell University

SLAYING THE FOOD MYTHS

THE TRUTH BEHIND THE HEADLINES

DR. STEVE CHANEY, PhD

ISBN: 978-1-64184-999-9

Book design by JETLAUNCH.net

About The Author

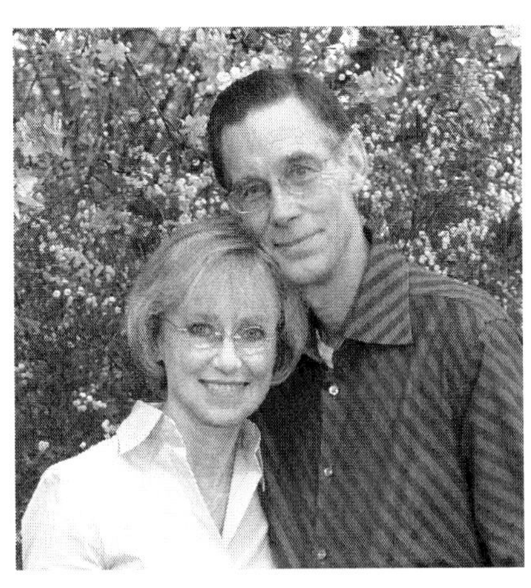

Dr. Steve Chaney received his B.S. degree in Chemistry from Duke University and his Ph.D. degree in Biochemistry from UCLA. He is currently Professor Emeritus at the University of North Carolina at Chapel Hill. At the time of his retirement he held the title of Distinguished Professor in the Department of Biochemistry and Biophysics and the Department of Nutrition.

Dr. Chaney is an educator who taught human metabolism and nutrition to first year medical and dental students for 40 years. He was named "Basic Science Teacher of the

Year" several times by the first-year medical students and was awarded the "Excellence in Teaching Lifetime Achievement Award" by the Academy of Educators upon his retirement in 2012.

Dr. Chaney is a scientist who ran an active cancer research program for 37 years. He was internationally known for his research on the biochemistry of anticancer drugs. He helped develop a drug that represents a major advance in the treatment of colon cancer and was a featured speaker at 6 international symposia on anticancer drugs.

Dr. Chaney is an author who has published over 100 papers and 12 reviews in peer-reviewed scientific journals as well as two chapters on nutrition for the first 6 editions of one of the leading biochemistry textbooks for medical students. Dr. Chaney is committed to helping people lead healthier lives and is highly sought after as a speaker on the topic of holistic approaches to health.

In his 40 years of teaching medical students and public speaking, Dr. Chaney realized just how confusing nutrition was to the average person. One day saturated fat is going to kill you. The next day it's good for you. Diets range from Jack Sprat "who could eat no fat" to his wife "who could eat no lean". Myths are repeated so many times people believe they must be true.

Dr. Chaney realized that people needed an accurate source of nutrition information they could trust. So, he founded his https://healthtipsfromtheprofessor.com weekly blog upon his retirement from the University of North Carolina. His mission is to cut through the hype and urban myths to provide you with the truth about how you can attain and maintain optimal health. He created his blog and has written this book because people like you need resources they can rely on for up-to-date, scientifically accurate health information without hype or bias. His goal is to provide you with accurate health information based on the latest clinical studies and to help you avoid the sensational and misleading claims in the media.

Foreword

Considering my early years, I might be considered the least likely person to be writing a book about nutrition and health, particularly one that features the myths about healthy foods and a healthy diet.

Growing up, I ate a typical American diet. My mother believed in a balanced diet – as long as it came from a can or a box. My father prided himself on being able to grill the perfect steak. Salads were often a canned pear in lime Jello, served on iceberg lettuce with a dollop of Cool Whip on top. Of course, if you cleaned your plate, there was always dessert. I quickly learned to eat everything on my plate, whether I liked it or not. We didn't drink sodas with meals, but there were plenty of sodas, chips and sweets on hand for between meals. As a teenager, my favorite places to eat were Amado's Pizza and the Charburger Grill (the name says it all).

In my 20s, I never thought much about nutrition, or that what I ate could affect my health. I never thought about supplementation. After all, my mother had taught me that my "balanced diet" would provide everything I needed. As a college student, I often got colds. I was usually tired by mid-afternoon. I thought that was normal. After all, I was a typical student. I kept crazy hours. I just needed an over-the-counter cold medicine and more coffee.

In graduate school my life started to change. I met my beautiful and amazing soulmate, Suzanne. She had been raised by a mom who believed in natural, holistic approaches to health – including a healthy diet and supplementation. By the standards of her time, her mom was a "health nut." Actually, she was way ahead of her time.

It turns out that one of the most valuable lessons my mother taught me was: "never argue with the cook." I didn't have to eat what she cooked for dinner, but there were no substitutes. Her saying was "If you don't eat your dinner, breakfast is in the morning." There were no after dinner snacks. When Suzanne and I got married, her cooking was very different from what I was used to. There were vegetables I had never heard of. Meat was no longer the centerpiece of every meal. I was eating more oatmeal & bran cereal and less eggs & bacon. Desserts often became fresh fruit instead of cakes, pies and cookies. However, because of what my mother had taught me, I just ate what Suzanne cooked. I was eating healthier, but I never thought about it. It was not a conscious decision on my part.

I don't want you to think that my diet became perfect the moment I married Suzanne. It was still an evolution. In our early years, we bought a quarter of a cow at a time and stored the meat in a freezer locker. That meant we were eating a lot of beef in those days. Suzanne also had a family recipe for cheese pie (cream cheese, sour cream, and lots of sugar) that was "to die for." However, the more we learned about nutrition and health the more our diet changed. The servings of meat got smaller and smaller. Beef was replaced with chicken and fish. Meat went from being the centerpiece of our meals to a garnish. The cheese pie became a fond memory.

I also wouldn't want you to think that my nutrition education was instantaneous. Encouraged by my mother-in-law, I began to investigate the impact of diet on health outcomes. My mother-in-law encouraged me to read Organic Gardening and various health magazines in addition to the scientific literature I was reading for my graduate courses. Of course, I didn't automatically believe everything I read in those magazines. As a graduate student, I was a "skeptic in training." I checked out what those magazines had to say by reading the pertinent scientific literature. I rejected a lot of what I read, but some of it rang true. Little by little I learned how important good nutrition and a healthy lifestyle were to my overall health. More importantly, I learned how to separate fact from fiction.

The changes in diet and lifestyle that I have made over the years have paid off. I am now in my 70s and am in perfect health, with no illnesses and no medications. As I look back, I wish I could have told my younger self what I know now. More importantly, I want to share this information with so many young people who, like my earlier self, know nothing about nutrition and how important it is to their health. After all, most of them will not be fortunate enough to marry someone who cares as much about healthy eating as my wife. They won't have a mother-in-law to guide them along the path to good health. I want these young people to enjoy the same health when they reach their golden years as I enjoy today. I also realized how hard it is for the average person to sort through the myths about healthy foods and diet that abound in today's world. I want to give people a guide, so they can cut through the misinformation and discover the truth about healthy eating. That is the genesis of this book, **"Slaying the Food Myths."**

In addition to cooking nutritious meals, my wife put a multivitamin by my plate every day. I didn't think much about it. I just considered it part of the meal and took it (remember my mother's rule: "Never argue with the cook"). I started to feel better. I had more energy. I had fewer colds. That roused my curiosity. Could that multivitamin actually have made a difference? Remember, I was a "skeptic in training." I knew about the placebo effect. I started scanning the scientific literature, so I could separate fact from fiction about supplementation. I learned that, under the appropriate conditions, supplementation was effective. I also learned that there was a lot of hype and misinformation about supplementation. That is the genesis of my upcoming book, **"Slaying the Supplement Myths."**

As I was learning about supplementation, I assumed that the FDA regulated the supplement industry in the same way it regulated the drug industry. As I learned more, I was horrified to find out that was not the case. Quality controls were not required. While a few companies were making high quality supplements, many companies were not. They had no quality controls. You had no idea what you were getting. Their products might have little or no active ingredients. They might have impurities. They might even have dangerous contaminants.

I also assumed that the FDA must surely require supplement manufacturers to conduct clinical studies proving that their products were safe and effective. Once again, I was sorely disappointed. The FDA did not require proof of safety and efficacy in the supplement industry.

When you think about it, this is the worst of all possible worlds. There are supplements on the market with no quality controls and no proof that they work. Yet if you look at their literature, it sounds like these supplements are as pure as the driven snow and can cure all your ills. What I have learned about the dark side of the food supplement industry is the basis for section 1 of "Slaying the Supplement Myths." I call that section: "**The Lies of the Charlatans**."

Like everyone else, I was also confused by all the conflicting headlines about supplementation in my younger years. One day you were told nutrient "X" would cure you.

The next day you were told it would kill you. Over my 40 years of scientific research I became quite skilled at analyzing the strengths and weaknesses of scientific publications. Eventually, I started to use these skills to analyze the publications behind the headlines, so I could determine which of them were bogus and which were true. The more I learned, the more I wanted to share this information with others. I knew the conflicting headlines must be just as confusing to others as they had been for me. You will find that information in section 2 of "Slaying the Supplement Myths." I call that section: "**The Myths of the Naysayers**."

Dr. Steve Chaney, PhD

P.S. In addition to these books I have created a weekly blog called "Health Tips From the Professor" (https://healthtipsfromtheprofessor.com). Each week I start with a recent headline, analyze the study behind the headline, and give a balanced, scientifically sound evaluation of the claim(s) made in the headline. I tell you whether you should ignore the headline or act on it. In addition, I have started providing educational Facebook Live videos on my Steve Chaney Facebook page.

Acknowledgements

I would like to start by acknowledging my beautiful wife Suzanne who has put up with a skeptical professor and kept him healthy all these years. They say that "Behind every successful man there is a good woman." I would reword that to say: "Behind every healthy man there is a wise woman." However, Suzanne is much more than that. She is my companion and soulmate. She is also very successful in her own right.

I would like to acknowledge my mother-in-law, Mary Becker, who was my inspiration and my guide. I would like to acknowledge my son Marc, who encouraged me to write this book. Finally, I would like to acknowledge my daughter-in-law, Ashley. Marc and Ashley already know much more about nutrition than I did at their age and are raising our granddaughter, Kaziah Grace, with love and good nutrition.

Disclaimer

The statements in this book have not been approved by the Food and Drug Administration. They are not intended to diagnose, treat, cure, or prevent disease. More importantly, the information in the book is not meant to replace the advice of your health professional. Rather, it is meant to be something you discuss with your health professional as you partner together to create your healthy living plan.

Table Of Contents

Overview

Knowledge is power! This book is unlike any other diet book you have ever read. Most diet books are written by some self-proclaimed diet guru. They are based on the premise that only the author knows the "truth." He or she knows the perfect diet to help you lose weight and live a long and healthy life. The purpose of their book is to convince you that they are right and to give you guidelines for following their "perfect diet."

I will make recommendations about foods, supplements, and diets when I think they are based on good science. But the real purpose of this book is to give you, my readers, the knowledge you need to become more informed consumers. I can only point out the fads and follies that exist today. You will need the knowledge to recognize those that will arise in the future.

I will debunk the myths and misleading information that are so prevalent in the nutrition sphere today. I will also point out the weaknesses in some of the studies that back truly healthy foods and diets. In the process I hope to teach you how to view each new diet pronouncement with healthy skepticism. I hope to teach you how to separate the "wheat from the chaff." If I have achieved that goal for any of you, I will have armed you to avoid the pitfalls and wayward paths along your quest for better health. I will have empowered you to make healthy choices today and in the future. I will consider this book a success.

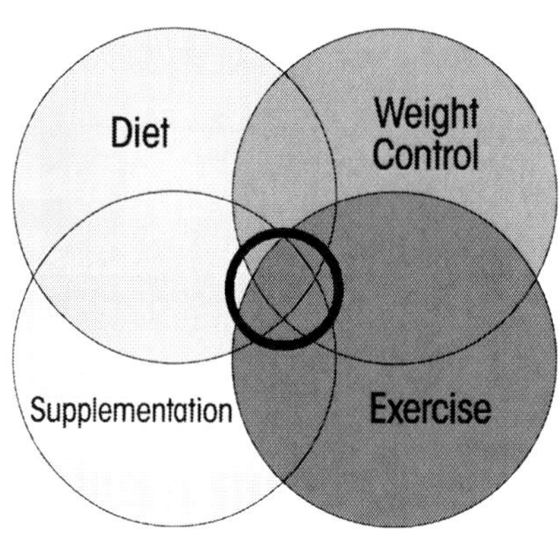

To help orient you to the themes of this book I have created a graphic for holistic living that I call "A Design For Healthy Living." This graphic is designed to make the point that a holistic lifestyle includes a healthy diet, a healthy weight, exercise, and appropriate supplementation. Of course, the sweet spot is that red circle in the middle.

In this book I cover healthy foods and a healthy diet and in some detail. I also orient you to the proper role of supplementation in a healthy diet. In my upcoming book, "Slaying the Supplement Myths", I will cover the pros and cons of supplementation so that you can become more informed consumers of supplements as well. Weight control deserves a whole book of its own. Perhaps I may be inspired to write that book someday.

Finally, I recognize that exercise, adequate sleep, proper hydration, stress reduction, spirituality, community and many other factors are also part of a healthy lifestyle. For those aspects of holistic living I turn you over to other authors who have made them their life's work. That is because I know my strengths and weaknesses. I have spent a lifetime studying and teaching human metabolism and nutrition. That is my expertise. I choose not to offer opinions in areas where I am less informed.

I could have subtitled this book "The Great American Food Fight" because almost everything we thought we knew about healthy foods and a healthy diet has become controversial. More importantly, these controversies have become like the global warming debate. There are camps on either side of every issue who are absolutely convinced they are right and absolutely convinced that the other side is wrong. It has become a "food fight." Science and rational thought have gone out the window. I hope to reintroduce them into the discussion with this book.

What I Wish I'd Known At 20

I was a typical 20-year-old American. I ate lots of junk food. I thought an occasional tennis game was all the exercise I needed. I never really thought about what I was doing. I just did what my friends did. If I hadn't changed what I was doing, I might have had a short, unhealthy life.

Of course, I did change, and those changes made all the difference. Now I'm in my 70s, and I'm in perfect health. I have no diseases. Even the allergies I had when I was younger have gone away as I improved my diet and lifestyle. I am on no medications. I have the blood pressure of a 16-year-old.

I call this introduction "What I Wish I'd Known At 20," but this isn't just about me. I wrote this for all the other 20-year-olds who know as little about nutrition and health as I did at 20. I also wrote this article for all those people who haven't changed – those people with the same diet and lifestyle they had at 20. It's never too late to change.

15 "Secrets" I Learned Along The Way

Here are 15 tips I would pass along to all the 20-year-olds, even those 20-year-olds in older bodies:

#1: You Are In Charge, Not Your Doctor: You have a brain. You have free will. You don't have to do what everyone else is doing. It is time to start thinking about what your health and your life will be like if you don't change. More importantly, it is time to start thinking about what your health and your life could be like if you do make positive changes.

#2: It Matters: I can't emphasize strongly enough how important it is to make positive changes in your diet, your exercise, and your overall lifestyle. We know all the major killer diseases (heart disease, cancer, diabetes and hypertension) are affected by diet and lifestyle. However, it is much more than avoiding disease. As you age, your quality of life is dramatically affected by how much you have moved and what you have put in your mouth over your lifetime.

#3: Avoid the Fads: Once you have decided to adopt a healthier lifestyle, the hardest part is deciding which changes you should make. You will need to practice a lot of due diligence. There is a lot of hype and misinformation out there. There is a new fad every week. First, it's low-fat. Then it's low-carb. Then it's no bananas before noon on Thursdays. (I'm joking here, but you get the point. Some of the diets are just plain weird.)

Most of those diet recommendations sound plausible. They all have their advocates who are only too happy to offer their testimonials. My advice: If it sounds too good to be true, avoid it. If they tell you the medical profession is trying to keep their diet a secret, avoid it. The consensus advice of the medical and nutrition communities may seem boring, but it is generally based on dozens of clinical studies. It is much more likely to be true than advice from your friends, your trainer, or that blogger who values controversy more than accuracy.

#4: We Are All Different: Health recommendations are usually based on dozens of clinical studies. But here is the "secret" you may not have known. Clinical studies report averages, but none of us are average. Let me give you an example. Let's say you wanted to do a clinical study to evaluate whether a low-carb diet helps people lose weight. You might enroll several hundred people in your study. If you put them all on an identical low-carb diet for 8 weeks, some of them would lose weight. Others would gain weight. At the end of the 8 weeks, you would average all weight changes together and report the average weight loss.

For the sake of argument, let's say the average weight loss was 6.4 pounds. That's fine except that not a single person in the study lost exactly 6.4 pounds, and some may have even gained weight. The bottom line is that your results may be different from conventional wisdom. Your results may be different from your friend's. You will need to find out what works best for you.

#5: You Don't Have To Change All At Once: Some people have an iron will and can make drastic changes overnight. Most of us aren't like that. If we try to change too many things at once, we become overwhelmed. We become discouraged. Sometimes we quit. Think of this as a marathon, not a sprint. Make "Change One Thing At A Time" your mantra. Change one thing each week until you are where you want to be. One week it may be replacing sugary desserts with fruits. Another week it may be adding a green vegetable to your dinner plate. Over time, all those small changes will result in a totally different lifestyle.

#6: Your Tastes Will Change: The first time you choose a low sodium food, it will taste bland. Over time you will come to enjoy the subtle flavors of the food and will come to dislike added salt. The first time you switch from whole milk to low-fat milk it will taste like water. Over time you will learn to appreciate low-fat milk, and whole milk will taste greasy. I could give lots more examples, but you get the point.

#7: Processed Foods, Sweets, and Sodas Will Kill You: I'm being dramatic here, but virtually all health experts agree that they are bad for your health. They have no place as part of a healthy diet. Replace the processed foods and sweets with whole foods. Replace the sodas with water or herbal teas.

#8: It's What You Do Every Day That Matters: Refined grains, pastries and sweets should be only an occasional indulgence. Fruits, vegetables, whole grains, nuts, beans and seeds should be the mainstay of your everyday diet. Eat a plant-based diet as much as possible.

#9: Protein Is Important, Especially As We Get Older: Low-fat or vegetarian protein sources should be your first choice. Chicken (with the skin removed) and fish are the healthiest meats. Nuts, beans and seeds are excellent vegetarian protein sources, especially in combination. Think of red meats as no more than an occasional indulgence.

#10: Avoid The Center Of The Supermarket: This is my only shopping advice. In general, supermarkets are arranged with real foods around the edges and processed foods in the middle. Of course, supermarkets know the shopping patterns of health-conscious people and will try to trick you into buying higher profit unhealthy foods. For example, our local markets place Cool Whip and sugar cakes next to the strawberries in the spring.

#11: Choose Organic: Our planet has become so polluted that is has become almost impossible to completely avoid toxic chemicals in our environment. They are in our air, our water, our soil, and our homes. Our only defense is to be informed consumers and avoid them whenever possible. If the cost of organic produce is an issue for you, be selective. If you do a quick internet search, you will find a "Dirty Dozen" list of fruits and vegetables that are the ones most likely to be contaminated with pesticides and herbicides. Those fruits and vegetables will be the best use of your organic spending allowance.

#12: Get Lots Of Exercise: Most experts recommend at least 30 minutes of moderate intensity exercise 5 times per week. More is even better. For best results choose a combination of aerobic and weight bearing exercise.

#13: Control Your Weight: We are in the midst of an obesity epidemic. The problem is that 80% of us are genetically predisposed to become obese if we eat a typical American diet and follow a typical American lifestyle. The solution isn't the fad diet du jour. The solution is to change our diet and our lifestyle. For most of us, the changes I outlined in this book will allow you to gradually attain and maintain your ideal weight.

#14: Supplementation Plays A Role: Supplementation is not a magic bullet, but it is an important component of a holistic wellness program. Some of us need supplementation to fill in nutritional gaps in our diet. Some of us need supplementation because of increased needs, diseases, or genetics. Some of us choose supplementation to achieve optimal health.

#15: Enjoy The Journey: If you think of a healthy lifestyle as depriving you of the things you enjoy, you will avoid it. Instead, think of it as an adventure. Have fun exploring new fruits and vegetables. Try cooking with herbs and spices. Seek out restaurants and recipes that turn healthy foods into a gourmet experience. Find exercises that you enjoy.

1

Why Is Optimal Nutrition So Important?

I could begin by repeating what every other diet book you have read has probably told you already. I could tell you that if you don't clean up your diet, control your weight, and get off the couch, you are doomed to a short, unhealthy life. You are likely to be cut down at an early age by heart disease, stroke or cancer. If you do reach your golden years, they will be anything but golden. All of that is true, but I'm not going to talk about it. Instead, I'm going to give you some reasons for making healthy lifestyle changes that you may not have heard before.

Our Mighty Microbiome And Our Health

When you read that title, you probably had three questions:

1) What is our microbiome?
2) How is it affected by our diet?
3) What does it have to do with our health?

Let me start at the beginning. The term ***microbiome*** refers to all the microorganisms in the human body. For our purposes, microbiome refers primarily to intestinal microorganisms. Most of you probably already know about the concept of "good" and "bad" intestinal microorganisms. Evidence suggests that the "bad" bacteria and yeast in our intestines can cause all sorts of adverse health effects:

- There is mounting evidence that they can compromise our immune system.
- There is also evidence that they can create a "leaky gut" (you can think of this as knocking holes in our intestinal wall that allow partially digested foods to enter the circulation where they can trigger inflammation and auto-immune responses).
- There is some evidence that they can affect brain function and our moods.
- They appear to convert some of the foods that we eat into cancer-causing chemicals which can be absorbed into the bloodstream.
- Studies in mice even suggest that they can make us fat.

"Good" bacteria, on the other hand, are thought to:

- Crowd out the "bad" bacteria and prevent many of the health problems they cause.

- Break down undigested fiber into beneficial end products like butyric acid, which is absorbed into the bloodstream and is thought to help regulate cholesterol and blood sugar levels.

In case you're thinking that it seems a bit far-fetched to believe that our intestinal bacteria could affect our health, let me remind you that we have about 39 trillion bacteria in our intestines compared to about 30 trillion cells in our body. They outnumber us.

The concept of "good" bacteria and "bad" bacteria has spawned the multimillion-dollar probiotics industry. Probiotics are based on a pretty simple concept. We have a few species of bad bacteria in our intestines. All we need to do is to replace them with a few species of good bacteria and we will be healthier.

However, two recent discoveries have revolutionized our thinking about intestinal bacteria and our health.

#1: Our intestinal bacteria are incredibly diverse. Each of us has about 1,000 distinct species of bacteria in our intestines.

#2: The species of intestinal bacteria in our intestines are influenced by our diet.

I'm going to get a bit technical here. (Don't worry. There won't be a quiz.) Previous studies have shown that people from all over the world tend to have one of two distinct microbiomes (populations of microorganisms) in their intestines – Bacteroides or Prevotella. [Don't let the specialized scientific terminology scare you. These are just the names scientists have given to these two distinctive populations of intestinal bacteria.]

A recent study[1] showed that people who habitually consumed high-fat/low-fiber diets (diets containing predominantly animal protein, saturated fats, simple carbohydrates and sugar) tended to have the Bacteroides microbiome in their intestines, while people who habitually consumed low-fat/high-fiber diets (diets that are primarily plant-based and are high in complex carbohydrates and low in meat and dairy) tended to have the Prevotella microbiome in their intestines. And surprisingly this appears to be independent of sex, weight and nationality.

The research defining these two distinct microbiomes (populations of intestinal bacteria) and showing that they are influenced by what we eat is relatively new. At this point in time we know relatively little about the health benefits and risks associated with the Bacteroides and Prevotella microbiomes. For example:

- Most of the studies on the health effects of "bad intestinal bacteria" were based on the identification of one or two "bad bacteria" in the gut – not on the thousands of bacterial species found in the Bacteroides microbiome. So, we can't say for sure that the Bacteroides microbiome found in people with diets high in animal protein and saturated fats will cause the same health problems as the "bad bacteria" identified in earlier studies. Nor do we know for sure how important a role the Bacteroides microbiome plays in the health consequences of consuming that kind of diet.
- Similarly, many studies on the health benefits of "good intestinal bacteria" have been based on probiotic supplements containing one or two bacterial species – not the thousands of bacterial species found in the Prevotella microbiome. So, we can't really say if probiotics or even the Prevotella microbiome will convey the same health benefits seen in populations who consume vegetarian diets.

However, there are a few recent studies suggesting that our microbiomes are very important. Let me share one with you.

Carnitine and Heart Disease Risk

Perhaps I should start by giving you a little bit of background about carnitine. Carnitine is an essential part of the transport system that allows fatty acids to enter organelles called mitochondria in our cells. Mitochondria oxidize fatty acids and generate energy. So, carnitine is an essential nutrient for any cell that has mitochondria and utilizes fatty acids as an energy source.

Carnitine is particularly important for muscle cells, and the hardest-working muscle cells in our body are those that pump blood through our hearts. So, when we think of carnitine we should think of heart health first. But that doesn't mean that carnitine is an essential nutrient. In fact, our bodies generally make all the carnitine that we need. There are some metabolic diseases that can prevent us from making carnitine or utilizing carnitine efficiently. People with those diseases benefit from carnitine supplementation, but those diseases are exceedingly rare.

There is some evidence that supplemental carnitine may be of benefit in individuals suffering from congestive heart failure and other diseases characterized by weakened heart muscles. Other than that, there is little evidence that supplemental carnitine is beneficial for healthy individuals.

Considering the longstanding association between carnitine and heart health, you can imagine my surprise when I came across headlines a few years ago saying: "Cleveland Clinic study links L-carnitine to increased risk of heart disease." I decided to check it out. Here is what I found. In this study[2], the authors were trying to gain a better understanding of the well-established link between red meat consumption and cardiovascular disease risk. The classical explanation of this link has been the saturated fat and cholesterol content of the red meat.

However, several recent studies have questioned whether saturated fat and cholesterol actually increase the risk of cardiovascular disease (more about this later). Since red meat is also high in L-carnitine, the authors hypothesized that it might be the L-carnitine or a ***metabolite*** of the L-carnitine that was associated with increased risk of heart disease in people consuming red meat. The term metabolite refers to a small molecule that is either a breakdown product of something we eat or a building block for something the cell makes.

The authors homed in on a metabolite of L-carnitine called trimethylamine-N-oxide or TMAO that is produced by bacteria in the intestines and had been previously shown to accelerate atherosclerosis in mice. They developed what they called an L-carnitine challenge. Basically, they gave their subjects an 8-ounce sirloin steak, which contains about 180 mg of carnitine, and measured levels of carnitine and TMAO in the blood one hour later and in the urine 24 hours later. [I'm guessing they didn't have much trouble finding volunteers for that study.]

When the subjects were carnivores (meaning meat eaters) they found a significant increase in both carnitine and TMAO in their blood and urine following the L-carnitine challenge. When they put the same subjects on broad-spectrum antibiotics for a week to wipe out their intestinal bacteria and repeated he L-carnitine challenge, they found an increase in carnitine but no increase in TMAO. This simply confirmed that the intestinal bacteria were required for the conversion of carnitine to TMAO.

Finally, because previous studies have shown that carnivores and vegetarians have very different populations of intestinal bacteria, they repeated their L-carnitine challenge in a group of vegans and found that consumption of the same 8-ounce sirloin steak by the vegans did not result in any significant increase in TMAO in either their blood or urine.

Armed with this information, the authors measured carnitine and TMAO concentrations in the fasting blood of 2595 patients undergoing cardiac evaluation in the Cleveland Clinic. They used an established protocol to assess the three-year risk for major adverse cardiac events in the patients they examined. They observed a significant association between carnitine levels and cardiovascular event risks, but only in subjects who also had high blood levels of TMAO.

Now it's time to compare what the headlines said to what the study actually showed. The headlines said "L-carnitine linked to increased risk of heart disease." What the study showed was that there were two things that were required to increase the risk of heart disease – carnitine and a population of intestinal bacteria that converted the carnitine to TMAO.

The major source of carnitine in the American diet is red meat, and habitual red meat consumption is required to support a population of intestinal bacteria that convert carnitine to TMAO. So, the headlines should have read "red meat consumption linked to increased risk of heart disease." But of course, that's old news. It doesn't sell subscriptions.

This is one of dozens of recent studies suggesting that our microbiome affects how the foods we eat are metabolized in the intestines – sometimes with beneficial effects and sometimes with negative effects. However, microbiome research is in its infancy. We have much more to learn about how our diet affects our microbiome, and how our microbiome affects our health. Stay tuned.

Epigenetics: Can We Change Our Genetic Destiny?

When I was a young graduate student I read an article called "The Seventh Generation" in Organic Gardening magazine. That article was based on the old Indian admonition to consider the effects of everything we do on the seventh generation of our descendants.

The article was written before the environmental movement had co-opted the "seventh generation" concept. It was also written at a time when the food industry and the public had really started buying into the "better living through chemistry" concept. Processed foods, fast foods and artificial ingredients had just started to replace real foods in the American diet.

The author envisioned a world in which, if we continued to eat nutrient-depleted foods, each generation would be sicker than the previous generation until by the seventh generation our descendants would live miserable, sickly, shortened lives – and nobody would know why. The author did not have the foresight to predict the obesity epidemic, so he did not envision a world in which we might live sicker, shorter lives in as little as one or two generations.

In addition, the author was not a scientist, and his whole premise seemed scientifically implausible at the time. In those days, we thought that all genetic information resided in our DNA. During conception, we picked up some DNA from our dad and some from our mom, and that DNA was what made us a unique individual.

We knew that environmental influences such as diet, lifestyle and exposure to toxic chemicals could affect our health personally. However, we never dreamed that the effects of those environmental influences could alter our gene expression, and that those genetic alterations could be passed on to our children. Today we know that environmental influences can actually modify our DNA and that some of those modifications can be passed on to our offspring – a process called ***epigenetics***.

What Is Epigenetics And How Can It Affect Gene Expression?

Simply put, epigenetics involves modifications to our DNA. DNA can be methylated or acetylated, and the proteins that bind to our DNA can be modified in multiple ways. That is important for two reasons:

1) These alterations can turn genes on and off. That means that epigenetic modifications can alter gene expression.

2) These alterations can be influenced by our environment – diet, lifestyle, and exposure to environmental chemicals.

For example, one recent study[3] showed that 3 months of exercise was sufficient to change the methylation pattern of 5,000 genes in muscle cells. The change in methylation pattern activated genes involved in energy metabolism, improved insulin response, and reduced inflammation. Another study[4] showed that the changes in methylation pattern due to exercise activated genes that suppress cancer, and that this effect was most pronounced in older people. With respect to diet, a recent review[5] summarized studies showing that a variety of nutrients including folic acid, polyphenols, carotenoids, vitamin D and selenium influenced methylation patterns in tissues throughout the body. This review emphasized activation of genetically controlled pathways that suppress cancer, but other studies have suggested many other benefits of these nutrient-controlled alterations in gene methylation.

These findings raise the tantalizing question: Can we change our genetic destiny? For most of us, the answer appears to be a qualified yes. Let me share a few specific examples with respect to heart health.

- Perhaps the most impressive recent study[6] is one that looked at the effect of diet on 20,000 people who had a genetic predisposition to heart disease. These people all had a genetic variant 9p21 that causes a twofold increased risk of heart attack. The study showed that a diet rich in fruits, vegetables and nuts reduced their risk of heart attack to that of the general population.
- Another study[7], the Heart Outcomes Prevention Evaluation (HOPE) study, looked at genetic variations in the haptoglobin gene that influence cardiovascular risk. The haptoglobin 2-2 genotype increases oxidative

damage to the arterial wall, which significantly increases the risk of cardiovascular disease. When the authors of this study looked at the effect of vitamin E, they found that it significantly decreased heart attacks and cardiovascular deaths in people with the haptoglobin 2-2 genotype, but not in people with other haptoglobin genotypes.

- There was also a study called the ISOHEART study[8,9] that looked at a particular genetic variation in the estrogen receptor which increases inflammation and decreases levels of HDL. As you might expect, this genotype significantly increases cardiovascular risk. Soy isoflavones significantly decreased inflammation and increased HDL levels in this population group. But they had no effect on inflammation or HDL levels in people with other genotypes affecting estrogen reception.

These studies suggest that genetic predisposition [to heart disease] does not have to be your destiny. You can change the outcome. To put this into perspective, however, epigenetic studies are still in their infancy. We know you can influence your genetic destiny through diet and lifestyle. We know that diet and exercise cause epigenetic changes in our genome that influence pathways which are likely to reduce your risk of heart disease, diabetes, and cancer. What we do not yet have are long-term studies showing that those epigenetic changes influence health outcomes. Stay tuned. It will be fascinating to see what future research uncovers.

Even more monumental is the recent discovery that at least some epigenetic changes can be passed on to our children, which brings me to the question: "Can what we eat affect our kids?"

Animal Studies Showing Epigenetic Changes Can Be Inherited

As is often the case, the first definitive study showing that epigenetic changes were heritable was an animal study[10]. This study was done with a mouse strain called agouti. Agouti mice can have two remarkably distinctive phenotypes. They can either have a yellow coat, become obese as adults and be prone to cancer and diabetes as they age, or they can have a brown coat and grow up to be lean and healthy.

It had been known for some time that these phenotypic differences were controlled by the epigenetic methylation of a specific gene called the agouti gene. The agouti gene codes for a genetic regulator that controls coat color, feeding behavior, and body weight set-point, among other things. When the agouti gene is undermethylated it is active. Consequently, the mice have yellow coats and are prone to obesity. When the agouti gene is highly methylated it is inactive. The mice have brown coats and are lean and healthy. Moreover, methylation of the agouti gene is not a purely random event. Mothers with the yellow, obese phenotype tended to produce a preponderance of offspring with the same phenotype and vice versa. In short, the epigenetic methylation pattern of the agouti gene can be passed from generation to generation. It is heritable.

This study[10] broke new ground by showing that the methylation of the agouti gene could be strongly influenced by what the mother ate while the fetal mice were still in the womb. When the scientists fed agouti mothers a diet with extra folic acid, B12, betaine and choline (all nutrients that favor DNA methylation) during conception and pregnancy, the agouti gene of their offspring became highly methylated. A high percentage of those offspring had brown coats and grew up to be lean and healthy. However, when the scientists put agouti mothers on a diet that was deficient in folic acid, B12, betaine and choline during conception and pregnancy, the agouti gene of their offspring was undermethylated. Many of those offspring had yellow coats and grew up to be fat and unhealthy.

Subsequent studies from the same laboratory have shown that:

- Addition of genistein, a phytonutrient from soy, to the maternal diet also favors methylation of the agouti gene and protects against obesity in agouti mice[11].
- The addition of the environmental toxin bisphenol A to maternal diets causes undermethylation of the agouti gene and predisposes to obesity in agouti mice, but this effect can be reversed by also feeding the mother genistein or folic acid and related nutrients during pregnancy[12].

The agouti mice studies provide a dramatic example of how diet and environmental exposure during pregnancy can cause epigenetic changes in fetal DNA that have long-term health consequences for the offspring. However, they are animal studies. Does the same hold true for humans?

Human Studies Showing Epigenetic Changes Can Be Inherited

With humans, it is very difficult to determine whether epigenetic changes that occur during conception and pregnancy affect our children. That is because when you measure an epigenetic effect in a child or adult, it is difficult to sort out how much of that effect was caused by what the mom ate during pregnancy and how much was caused by how the family ate as the kids were growing up.

Unfortunately, there is a tragic human experiment that shows that the same kind of epigenetic changes are heritable in humans. I'm referring to what is known as the "Dutch Hunger Winter." This was a period of starvation during 1944-1945, the final year of World War II, when the Germans set up a blockade that prevented food from reaching western

Holland. During those few months, even pregnant women were forced to live on food rations providing as little as 500 calories a day.

This was an event without parallel in human history. Holland is not a third world country. Once the blockade was lifted, children born during the Hunger Winter had the same plentiful supply of food as every other Dutch citizen. This has allowed generations of research scientists to ask what were the effects of a brief exposure to malnutrition during conception and pregnancy.

The health consequences were dramatic. Fifty years later, individuals who were conceived during the Hunger Winter weighed about 14 pounds more, had waists about 1.5" larger, and were three times more likely to have heart disease than those born to mothers who were in their second or third trimester of pregnancy during that time. By the time they reached age 63, they experienced a 10% increase in mortality.

What caused those health consequences? Could the cause have been epigenetic? Research suggests that the answer might be yes. A recent study[13] analyzed epigenetic changes in DNA from blood samples of survivors born during the Hunger Winter that had been collected when they were 59 years old. This study showed:

- A distinct pattern of DNA methylation was observed in survivors who were conceived during the Hunger Winter. This pattern of DNA methylation was not observed in survivors whose mothers were in their second or third trimester during the Hunger Winter. It was also not seen in people who were conceived immediately before or after the Hunger Winter.

- Some of the genes with distinctive methylation patterns were genes that affected things like cholesterol levels and insulin sensitivity, which have the potential to increase disease risk.

- Other genes with distinctive methylation patterns were genes that affected metabolism. They were "thrifty" genes that increased the efficiency of metabolism. Increased efficiency of metabolism is beneficial when calories are scarce, but can lead to obesity when calories are plentiful.

That is a truly remarkable finding when you think about it. These data suggest that starvation during conception or early pregnancy caused the fetus to make epigenetic changes to its DNA that allowed it to become more efficient at energy utilization, and those epigenetic changes have lasted a lifetime – even when food was abundant throughout the rest of that lifetime.

There are many other examples of heritable epigenetic modifications. For example:

- When female rats are maintained on a "junk-food diet" high in fat and sugar during pregnancy and lactation their offspring show a marked preference for high fat foods[14]. They also show epigenetic alterations of the central reward pathways that may pre-condition them to require higher intakes of fat to experience pleasure from eating.
- When rats are fed diets deficient in omega-3 fatty acids, adolescent rats from the second and subsequent generations display marked increases in hyperactivity and anxiety[15], symptoms similar to human adolescents with ADHD.
- In a clinical trial of 162 obese Canadian mothers who had children before and after weight loss surgery, the children born after weight loss surgery were half as likely to grow up overweight or obese as the children born before the weight loss surgery[16], and this correlated with epigenetic modification of genes that play a role in obesity, diabetes, cancer and heart disease[17].

Taken together, the existing data suggest that our diet and environmental exposure during conception and pregnancy can cause epigenetic changes to our children's DNA that may affect their future health in ways that we can only begin to understand at present. It is a sobering thought. The "Seventh Generation" warning I read about in my youth may be real.

2

Why Is Nutrition So Confusing?

Hopefully you now have a better understanding of why diet, weight control, exercise, and other lifestyle choices are so important. The way we treat our bodies has a powerful effect on our health and longevity in ways that we are just beginning to understand. It can trump our genetics. More importantly, if what we are starting to learn about epigenetics is correct, the choices we make today can influence the health of our children, and maybe even our grandchildren. That makes our lifestyle choices an awesome responsibility.

The difficult part starts the moment you have decided that you will make healthier lifestyle choices. Should you go low fat or low carb? Should you eat all the saturated fats you want, or should you avoid them? Should you go vegan or Paleo or keto? Which weight loss program will give you the best long-term results? Should you focus on endurance exercises or weight training?

The headlines don't help. One week you will see headlines promoting a particular diet or health practice. The next week you'll see headlines telling you that doesn't work. You can find websites or blogs, some written by doctors, promoting different viewpoints, and most of them list scientific studies "proving" they are right. All of them can't be correct!

You just want to do the right thing. You just want to create better health for you and your children. But where do you start? Why does it have to be so confusing? This chapter is designed to help you understand the source of this confusion, so you can start to make better choices about which headlines and which websites to believe.

Secrets Only Scientists Know

You generally think of scientists as completely impartial, and we do our best to be. But you need to know that when we design a study, we do have an agenda. We're trying to disprove the generally accepted truths (often referred to as ***paradigms***). There is no glory in being the 10th person to prove a paradigm correct. The glory comes from disproving a paradigm that everybody else thought was true and establishing a new paradigm in the process.

Experiments Are Designed To Give Conflicting Results

Because of that we design our experiments to disprove what everyone else accepts as true. Of course, we all have our pet hypothesis, so our agenda is to disprove everyone else's hypotheses and prove our own hypothesis. I don't want to give you the idea that scientists are contrary. The fact that we set out to disprove each other's hypotheses is the real strength of the scientific method. It is through this constant testing and revaluation of the scientific literature that we ultimately arrive at the truth.

Now that you understand the agenda behind our experiments, you can better understand why the results of individual studies are often contradictory. They are designed to be contradictory. As scientists we expect that. When we scientists evaluate conflicting studies, we can sometimes figure out the reasons behind the differences. Sometimes it's because the study design is different. Sometimes it's because the population groups are different. But, quite often, we never really know why one study may say vitamins work, and another study may say they don't. That's why we never base our opinions on a single study. We base our opinions on multiple studies, something we refer to as the "weight of available evidence."

What I Learned As A Cancer Scientist

Another secret that only scientists seem to appreciate is that not all studies are created equal. Some carry far more weight than others. I was involved in cancer drug development for most of my 40-year research career. In developing a cancer drug, we evaluated potential drug candidates by sequentially moving them through are series of test tube studies, cell culture studies, animal studies, and human clinical trials. That experience has given me a unique insight into the relative value of various kinds of studies in predicting health outcomes.

Test tube studies generally involve looking at whether some compound can carry out a particular reaction or inhibit a particular enzyme. This kind of study is what we call "Proof of Principle." This just tells us whether the reaction or effect is feasible. In cancer research, we might start with 1000 candidate cancer drugs that looked feasible in the test tube.

The next step in the drug development process is to test the candidate drugs in **cell culture**. Many of them flunk out at this step. Some are not taken up by the cells. Some degrade rapidly once they enter the cell. Others simply do not work at a cellular level. Of the 1,000 candidate drugs from test tube studies, only about 100 work in living cells.

If they work at a cellular level, they are sent off to laboratories that specialize in **animal studies**. Once again, most of them don't make the cut. Some never make it into the bloodstream. Some are eliminated by the kidney or metabolized by the liver before they can make it to their target tissues. Of those 100 candidates that look promising in cell culture, only 10 work in animals.

If a candidate drug passes all those tests, it enters **human clinical trials**. Human metabolism and physiology is not identical to that of the mice and rats used in animal studies. Most of the remaining candidate drugs fail here. Of those 1,000 candidate drugs you started with, only one may make it into the clinic. That is if you are lucky. I was fortunate enough to have one of the compounds I worked on in my 40-year research career make it into the clinic. Many of my colleagues were not that fortunate. They made major contributions to science, but never had the satisfaction of seeing those contributions lead to a therapeutic intervention that saved lives.

Why do I mention this? Many of the headlines you see, or references you see cited in websites and blogs promoting a particular diet or supplement, are based on cell culture or animal studies. I want you to understand the relative predictive power of those studies. There is about a 10% chance that the findings of an animal study will apply to humans and about a 1% chance that the findings of a cell culture study will apply to humans. Unless the conclusions of cell culture and animal studies are validated by well-designed clinical studies, I would ignore them.

That, of course, brings me to the next source of confusion. This is another secret that only scientists seem to know. There are different kinds of clinical studies, and they don't all have the same predictive power.

Association Studies Versus Intervention Studies

In an ***intervention clinical study,*** you start with a group of people and divide them into two matched groups. One group is given a drug, or a supplement, or placed on a particular diet (the intervention). The other group serves as a control. (For drugs and supplements, the Gold standard study is double-blind, placebo controlled. That simply means neither the subject nor the investigators know who is receiving the intervention and who is serving as a control. Of course, double-blind studies are virtually impossible when the intervention is a diet.) Because dietary intervention studies are expensive, many dietary comparisons are what we call association studies.

There are two types of ***association clinical studies***. In one type you start with a group of people who follow a particularly diet and try to select a closely matched population group that does not and compare health outcomes. In the other type, you start with a group of people and ask them to fill out a diet questionnaire. On the basis of the answers to the questionnaire you grade them on how closely they follow a particular diet. Then you compare health outcomes of people who habitually follow that diet and those who don't. In either case you are looking at the association of health outcomes with adherence to a particular diet.

A lot of what we know about diet and lifestyle is based on association studies. These studies have provided many valuable insights, but they do have a significant weakness. Scientists call it a ***confounding variable***, but for clarity's sake I will refer to it as unintended associations. Simply put, the people adhering to a particular diet may being doing something else the investigators did not measure, and it is responsible for the health benefits associated with the diet. Perhaps they exercise more or see the doctor more often. It could be almost anything. The best of the association studies try to account for as many unintended associations as possible, but you can never be absolutely sure that they accounted for all of them.

I will give you a somewhat humorous example of association studies gone awry when I discuss chocolate consumption and weight loss in the chapter on Food Myths.

Every Clinical Study Has Its Flaws

Another secret that only scientists seem to know is that every clinical study has its flaws. Because of that, there is no one perfect clinical study that absolutely proves or disproves a hypothesis. Sometimes it could be the sample size, or the sample selection, that's flawed. Sometimes the control group was inappropriate. Sometimes the study is too short. Sometimes it is confounding variables – those unexpected things that influence the outcome. I'm going to give you some examples of each of those things in this book.

Statistics And Lies

Finally, there may also be problems with the statistical analysis. I love that quote from Mark Twain: "There are lies; there are damn lies and then there are statistics." Now don't get me wrong. There's not a scientist out there who tries to twist the statistical analysis to support their hypothesis. Well, maybe there are a few. But they are in the minority.

However, statistical analysis is a very complicated thing, and there are so many ways that it can mislead you. Because of that we can't just take statistical analyses at face value. We can't just say, "Oh, the statistics prove it." Sometimes we have to ask: "Is that logical?" "What do the other studies say?" "Is there a confounding variable that they overlooked?" You have to take statistics with a grain of salt.

What Good Scientists Do

I've given you all the dirty secrets about scientists, but a good scientist, at the end of the day, is going to be impartial. They'll be guided by the preponderance of published data. They don't go by a single study – even if it's their own study. A good scientist is constantly re-evaluating their hypotheses based on the latest studies. Good scientists readily admit when they are wrong. They are willing to discard their hypotheses when the data do not support them. That is the strength of the scientific method.

The problem is that many of the people who are providing you with diet and health information aren't scientists. They don't know the secrets that scientists know. With that in mind, let's look at where food myths come from.

Where Do Food Myths Come From?

Most food myths start with a blog or a website. Some of them are created by people with no training in nutrition or human metabolism. (I am always amazed that people with no training or knowledge of nutrition can create nutrition blogs that have millions of followers.) Some are created by medical doctors. Many of them are distinguished physicians, but there are things they do not know. They were probably never taught nutrition in medical school. They were not taught the scientific method, so they don't know "the secrets only scientists know." They were taught human metabolism in medical school, but it is what I refer to as "metabolism light." They were given an overview of human metabolism. There simply isn't time in the medical curriculum to take a deep dive into the details of metabolism.

They are all honorable people who start out with the best of intentions, but they are also intent on reaching lots of people. One way to create a large following in social media is to make your messages spectacular. It is the "man bites dog" stories that grab attention. Unfortunately, good science isn't always spectacular. Another way to create a large following is to grab people's attention by promising to reveal a truth that the medical community...or the scientific community...or the government...is hiding from you. The pressure to create a post that is spectacular AND grabs people's attention every week is immense. It is easy to see why some of these people "go over to the dark side."

I told you that good scientists look at the totality of research and rely on the weight of available evidence to drive their conclusions. Simply put, that means they base their conclusions on what the majority of good studies show. The "dark side" bloggers operate in reverse. They start with their bias and cherry pick the studies that support their bias, ignoring the rest. (Whether they do this on purpose or out of ignorance of the scientific method I do not know.) They then usually construct a metabolic rationale to support their conclusion based on what they remember from their biochemistry course in medical school. The results are often misleading at best and plain wrong at worst.

Once the initial blog post is published, social media takes over. The conclusions, right or wrong, are copied in blog after blog and website after website. It's akin to what we used to call a gossip chain in the old days. Once it has been repeated often enough that people start hearing it from multiple sources, it becomes generally accepted as true. Another food myth is born.

None Of Us Are Average

Another source of confusion is that dietary recommendations are based on clinical studies that report the average response to a particular diet. What if none of us are average? In fact, there is tremendous individual variability in how we respond to foods and to diets. Let me share two studies with you, one that shows the genetic potential for variability and one that shows just how large that variability can be.

Genetic Variation And You

We also know that family history is a strong predictor of genetic predisposition to disease. If you are a guy, and most of the males in your family tree have dropped dead of a heart attack at an early age, you can assume you are probably genetically predisposed to heart disease. If you are a gal and most of the women in your family tree have developed breast cancer at an early age, you can assume you are probably genetically predisposed to breast cancer.

However, if none of these apply, we assume we are "normal." We think we'll probably live to 120. All this healthy lifestyle "stuff" is nice, but it isn't a priority. It makes me think of Garrison Keillor's tales of "Lake Wobegon" where all the children were above normal. What if that weren't true? What if none of us are normal? What if all of us are predisposed to some disease, perhaps even multiple diseases, and don't know it? Would that change how we thought about making the effort to follow a healthy lifestyle?

A recent study[18] surveyed genomes of hundreds of individuals for loss of function (LOF) variants – mutations that would either partially or completely prevent the synthesis of a functional protein. After a very complex genetic analysis they concluded that each of us harbors about ~100 LOF variants in our genome.

Some of those mutations were in genes coding for proteins that have no known function. Other mutations coded for proteins whose loss might affect minor things like taste sensation. Still other mutations were in genes coding for proteins that were redundant because there are other proteins in the cell that can perform the same function. (Just as NASA designed the space shuttle with backup systems that could take over if a primary system failed, our bodies are often designed with more than one enzyme that can carry out the same function.)

However, the authors concluded that each of us harbors about 20 LOF mutations that completely inactivate essential genes and might increase the probability that we will develop certain diseases. That got me thinking. It validated scientifically something that we have all known instinctively for a long time – none of us are perfect. Or, as my childhood friends might have more cruelly put it: "We are all defective."

Now some of you may be saying: "What does this mean for me?" When you carry this idea through to its ultimate conclusion, the bottom line message is:

1) Conclusions from clinical trial results are based on averages – none of us are average.
2) Daily Values (DV) are based on averages – none of us are average.
3) Nutritional recommendations for optimal health are based on averages – none of us are average.
4) The identified risk factors for developing diseases are based on averages – none of us are average.

That means lots of the advice you may be getting about your risk of developing disease X, the best diet to prevent disease X, or the role of supplementation in preventing disease X may be generally true – but it might not be true for you.

So, my advice is not to blindly accept the advice of others about what is right for your body. Just because some health guru recommends it, doesn't mean it is right for you. Just because it worked for your buddy, doesn't mean it will work for you. Learn to listen to your body. Learn what foods work best for you. Learn what exercises just feel right for you. Learn what supplementation does for you.

Don't ignore your doctor's recommendations, but don't be afraid to take on some of the responsibility for your own health. You are a unique individual, and nobody else knows what it is like to be you.

Which Foods Lower Blood Sugar For You?

You may be wondering just how big individual variability is for things like diet. The answer is: "Pretty big." For example, there is lots of advice about foods that lower blood sugar on the internet. In a recent search, I found articles proclaiming "9 foods that lower blood sugar," "7 foods that control blood sugar," and "12 power foods to beat diabetes." But are those foods the right ones for you? What if we are remarkably different in our blood sugar responses to the same food? This is just what a recent study suggests.

A group of scientists in Israel[19] set out to test the hypothesis that people eating identical meals might have a high variability in their post-meal blood glucose response. Most previous studies have measured the average blood glucose response to various foods, and nutritional recommendations for which foods to eat when you are diabetic have been based on those studies. In this study, when the scientists measured average blood glucose responses to various foods, their results were identical to previous studies. However, when they looked at individual variation in blood sugar responses, their results were eye-opening.

For example, individual blood sugar responses varied:

- Four-fold for sugar-sweetened soft drinks, grapes and apples.
- Five-fold for rice.
- Six-fold for bread and potatoes.
- Seven-fold for ice cream and dates.

Put another way:

- Some people had almost no blood sugar response to cookies, but a very high blood sugar response to a banana.

- Other people had almost no blood sugar response to bananas, but a very high blood sugar response to cookies.

The authors concluded that "universal dietary recommendations [for lowering blood sugar levels] may have limited utility." That is because dietary recommendations are based on average responses and none of us are average. That is probably true of most other dietary recommendations as well. As the saying goes "We are all wonderfully [and differently] made."

So, when you read about diets and foods that will help you keep your blood sugar levels under control, take those recommendations with a grain of…sugar. They are a good starting place, but you need to listen to your body, and eat the foods that work best for you. Just don't get carried away, however. I'm pretty sure Twinkies washed down with a soft drink are bad for just about everyone.

That same advice is true for almost every other dietary recommendation you will hear. As I said earlier, it may be good for most people...it may have worked wonderfully well for your friend, but it might not be the right advice for you. You need to listen to your body. You need to ask yourself questions like: "What is my energy level?" "How do I feel?" "How is my digestion?" Weight loss, on the other hand, may not be the best measure because you can lose weight on an unhealthy diet (more about that later).

Big Food Inc Is Not Your Friend

Let's assume that you have cut through the myths and misinformation to find the perfect diet. You've experimented and found it is well suited for your body. There is one final trap that lies between you and optimal health – Big Food Inc. The big food companies are not your friends. They are not trusted companions on your quest for better health.

Big Food Inc follows the latest trends and are only too happy to give consumers what they want. You want low-fat? No problem. You want low-carb, natural, organic, non-GMO, gluten-free? No problem. However, their motive is a healthy bottom line, not your health.

They know humans are hardwired to desire sugar, salt, and fat. Foods with those ingredients sell. Convenience sells. At the end of the day, they are more interested in sales than they are health. They don't want you buying whole foods and cooking them from scratch. They want you to buy their pre-packaged convenience foods instead. Let's look at a few of the ways Big Food Inc tries to deceive you.

The Healthy Diet Hoax

The healthy diet hoax started back in the late 50s and early 60s when the American Heart Association started recommending a low-fat diet to reduce the risk of heart disease. Because fat is high in calories, other health organizations also recommended a low-fat diet for weight loss. What they envisioned was a diet with less fatty meats and dairy products, less processed foods, and more fruits, vegetables, legumes, and whole grains. However, that kind of change would have required people to change their food preferences and change their eating habits. It would also have cut into Big Food Inc's profits.

Big Food Inc immediately stepped in with a variety of "low-fat" processed and convenience foods. No need to change your eating habits. Just swap their "low-fat" processed foods for the processed foods you were already eating. These foods often contained fake fats – ingredients you would never find in real food – that gave their "low-fat" processed food the mouth feel and texture of the high fat food it was replacing. Even worse, to increase their consumer appeal these foods were often high in sugar, refined carbohydrates, and salt. These foods were even worse than the high fat foods they replaced.

They were junk foods masquerading as healthy foods because they could be labeled low-fat.

The consequences were predictable. The obesity epidemic continued unabated and heart disease remained our number one killer. That lead to the rise of the low-carb diet fad because "low-fat diets had failed." The irony is that it isn't the kind of low-fat diet envisioned by the American Heart Association that failed. That diet works quite well. It was Big Food Inc's version of the low-fat diet that failed.

Of course, Big Food Inc did not stop there. It has moved on to other popular diets as well. If the Atkins and South Beach diets ever had any possibility of being healthy, all hope was lost once Big Food Inc started to produce pre-packaged, convenient meals for people who wanted to follow those diets. Where will it end? I'm even starting to see pre-packaged Paleo meals in grocery stores.

Are Fast Foods Getting Healthier?

In recent months Panera, MacDonald's and Subway have all announced that they are switching to ingredients that people can recognize – ingredients that you might actually use in your own kitchen. Chipotle has recently announced that they have removed all genetically modified organisms from their foods. Pizza Hut said that it will remove artificial colors and preservatives from its food. Taco Bell pledged to remove artificial colors, artificial flavors, high-fructose corn syrup and palm oil from its foods.

For example, Taco Bell will start using real pepper instead of "black pepper flavor" in its food. (I didn't even realize that there was an artificial pepper flavor. Come on! Real pepper can't be that expensive!) They also plan to remove Yellow No. 6 from their nacho cheese, Blue No. 2 from their avocado ranch dressing, and carmine from their red tortilla strips.

Are fast foods getting healthier? Or is this all for show? Perhaps the first question to ask is: "Why is the fast food industry making these changes? Have they suddenly decided that they want to become part of the health food industry?"

One clue to those questions is the name of the parent company that owns both Pizza Hut and Taco Bell. They call themselves Yum Foods. You will notice that they don't call themselves Health Foods. Their name alone speaks volumes about their priorities. When the CEO of Yum Foods was describing these changes, he didn't speak about any desire to make the foods healthier. He spoke about responding to shifting consumer attitudes and the desire of consumers for "real food" as driving these kinds of changes. The bottom line is that fast food companies are realizing that consumers are becoming more aware of the dangers of artificial ingredients and are making their buying choices accordingly. The companies simply don't want to lose market share.

The second question to ask is: "Are these foods actually healthier?" The answer is: "Not really." None of these companies are talking about removing fat, sugar, salt or calories from their foods. They are more concerned with retaining the "yum" factor than they are in making their foods healthier.

Do You Want Hydrocolloids With That Pizza?

Even worse, some of the changes in the fast food industry are making their foods less healthy. Here the questions you should be asking are: "What is behind the curtain?" "What aren't they telling us about?" The answer is: "You probably don't want to know."

For example, I came across an interesting article in a food industry journal. A Spanish company called Premium Ingredients was announcing that they had developed a new "food" product from hydrocolloids and melting salts that could be used to replace casein in pizza toppings. [In case you were wondering, hydrocolloids are solids suspended in water to create a gel-like consistency (or in this case a cheese-like consistency), and melting salts are used as emulsifying agents to create a homogeneous product with extended shelf life.]

Now, a bit of background: You've heard nutritionists claim that pizza is a perfect food because it contains foods from all four food groups. Of course, that's ignoring the fact that pizza is generally made with white flour and contains lots of fat – mostly saturated fat, calories and sodium.

But when you look at many of the frozen and fast food pizzas on the market it gets even worse. Premium Ingredients didn't say that their hydrocolloids/melting salts mixture could be used to replace cheese. They said that it could be used to replace casein. That's because many pizza manufacturers haven't used real cheese in years. Instead they are using casein (a milk protein) and a chemical smorgasbord to manufacture a cheese "food" with the taste and consistency of cheese.

Cheese is a good source of protein and calcium, and it supplies a lot of other essential nutrients as well – such as vitamin D, vitamin A, vitamin B12, riboflavin, folic acid, magnesium and zinc. Some of the artificial cheeses on the market do supply the calcium found in real cheese, but almost none of them provide the other essential micronutrients. But, because the artificial cheeses have been made with casein up to now, we could at least count on them to supply the protein found in real cheese.

Now, thanks to Premium Ingredients, the manufacturers of frozen and fast food pizzas won't even have to use casein-containing artificial cheeses. In their trade journal article, Premium Ingredients boasted that their product will help manufacturers cut costs (and cut protein and essential nutrients in the process).

Lucky us! More and more artificial foods are coming on the market, and we have no idea what is in them.

Label Deception

Healthy Eating Is In. We are told we need more fiber, whole grains, fruits and vegetables, nuts, and omega-3s in our diet. Consequently, more and more Americans are reading food labels to be sure that the foods they are buying are healthy. But are those food labels deceptive? Is it possible that Big Food Inc could actually be lying to us? Once again, could it be that the food manufacturers care more about their profits than about our health?

For example, everyone knows that eating fiber-rich foods like fruits, vegetables, whole grains, and legumes is good for us. But wouldn't it be more fun if you could get the same amount of fiber in your breakfast bars, cakes, cookies and even yogurt?

The food manufacturers are only too happy to oblige. DuPont, for example, manufacturers an artificial fiber called Litesse by chemically linking glucose (dextrose) molecules into a non-digestible polydextrose polymer. They tell the food manufacturers that they can use Litesse to "tap into this market opportunity and project a healthier image for your product." I'd be much more impressed if they were talking about a healthier product rather than a "healthier image for your product." It's all about image, isn't it?

Similarly, Archer Daniels Midland manufactures a digestion-resistant form of maltodextrin they call Fibersol-2. They tell food manufacturers "Who knew fiber could be clean and clear?" (Translation: Adding bran to your products might make them denser and chewier. You can add Fibersol-2 to your doughnuts or cookies and it won't change their taste or texture).

The problem is that there are few clinical studies showing that these artificial fibers have the same benefits as the fibers we find in fresh fruits, vegetables and whole grains. In addition, these fibers don't fill you up the way that unprocessed fibers found in foods do (something we scientists refer to as satiety). For example, if you eat a bowl of oatmeal you're not going to be hungry for a long time. However, recent studies show that adding an equivalent amount of one of these artificial fibers to a muffin or breakfast bar has no effect on how hungry you feel after eating it.

Similarly, everyone knows that fruits and vegetables are good for us. They are chock full of vitamins, minerals, and phytonutrients as well as fiber. But who wants to spend the time peeling an orange or washing the pesticides off that broccoli? It's much more fun to get our fruits and vegetables from chips, pasta, and breakfast cereals.

Once again, the food manufacturers are only too happy to oblige. The chemical companies make a variety of fruit and vegetable powders that food manufacturers can add to their products. For example, PowderPure tells food manufacturers "Whether you want to add nutrition to your label, infuse full color, or formulate a specific flavor profile for your discerning consumers, PowderPure has the right powder to enhance your presence in the marketplace." You will notice they are talking about adding nutrition to the label, not to the food. They are talking about "enhancing your presence in the marketplace," not making your food healthier.

The problem is that sprinkling a little fruit and vegetable powder into a processed food will never provide the full range of nutrients that those fruits and vegetables would have provided. Most manufacturers can't (or won't) specify the amounts of nutrients and phytonutrients you get from the fruit and vegetable powders they add to their processed foods, but that doesn't stop them from making label claims like "We pop a flavorful blend of nine veggies...[in our chips]" or there is a "half serving of vegetables in a 2-oz serving…[of our pasta]."

My advice is to ignore the label claims of fruits and vegetables added to the processed foods you see in the market. The fruit and vegetable powders added to those foods provide no proven benefit. The best place to get your fruits and vegetables is to [surprise] eat your fruits and vegetables.

Summary: Cutting Through The Confusion

Now you know "the secrets that only scientists know," so you understand that not all scientific studies are reliable. You know how food myths are created, so you know to treat even widely held beliefs with skepticism. All of this has made you a more knowledgeable consumer of scientific information. You now understand that we are all different, so you realize that what works for other people may not work for you. Finally, you know that Big Food Inc is trying to lure you off the road to better health.

You now have the knowledge to cut through the confusing and often misleading information you find on the internet. Let's use that new-found knowledge to debunk some of the biggest food myths on the internet.

3

The Top 10 Food Myths Busted

It's time to tackle food myths and point out why they are so misleading. There are dozens of food myths, with new ones appearing every day, but I will limit myself to the top 10. Before I begin the process of busting popular food myths, let's consider how those myths arise in the first place.

How Do Food Myths Get Started?

Anything Is Better Than The Standard American Diet

Many of the myths that you hear arise from a misunderstanding or misrepresentation of what Americans are eating. For example, some people choose to focus on the refined carbohydrates and sugar in our diet. They will cite numerous studies showing that sugar consumption is associated with all the major diseases that afflict us. Other people choose to focus on the fat, especially saturated fat and trans fat, in our diet. They will quote numerous studies showing that fat consumption is associated with all the major diseases that afflict us. How can we reconcile such diametrically opposite viewpoints?

The key word here is "associated." Whenever you hear that word you need to ask: "What else might be associated with…?" It turns out that the American diet is high in both sugar and fat, and the two usually go hand in hand. There are relatively few foods that are just high in sugar. Sodas and sugar-sweetened juices are examples. We may think of pastries as sugar-rich foods, but your favorite cookie recipe probably contains a cup or more of both sugar and butter, or some other fat. There are also relatively few foods that are just high in fat. Butter, margarine and cream are examples. However, you will even find sugar in some salad dressings and some brands of peanut butter.

There are two important conclusions from the close association between fat and sugar in the American diet.

- A correlation between sugar intake and terrible health outcomes is not, in itself, sufficient to warrant a low-carb or a sugarless diet. Most of those people are also eating a lot of unhealthy fats. Similarly, a correlation between fat intake and terrible health outcomes is not, in itself, sufficient to warrant a low-fat diet. Most of those people are also eating a lot of sugar and unhealthy carbohydrates.
- Almost anything is better than the Standard American Diet. That is why proponents of even the most bizarre diets can make the claim that their diet is "healthy" (more about that later).

How did the American diet get so bad? There are two important reasons:

#1: We are hardwired to like foods that are high in sugar, salt and fat. When you think about it, those instincts were of great value when we were hunters and gatherers. Fruits are a great source of fiber, essential vitamins and phytonutrients, but in the wild fruits are scarce and seasonal. Our desire for sweet foods provided the incentive needed to search out fruits wherever we could find them. The story with salt is similar. We require a certain amount of salt in our diet, but it was a very scarce resource. In biblical times, salt was a valued commodity that was worth its weight in gold.

#2: The story with fat is a bit different. Our carbohydrate stores can fuel our body for only a day or two. Our protein stores can fuel our body longer, but we are cannibalizing essential proteins just to keep our body supplied with energy. Fat stores, on the other hand, can fuel our body for weeks or months. Thus, it only made sense to eat as much fat as possible when game was plentiful so that we would have sufficient fat stores to carry us through times of scarcity.

These instincts served us well when we were hunters and gatherers, but work to our disadvantage in a society in which food is plentiful 24/7. The bad news is that the more we eat foods that are high in sugar, salt, and fat, the more we crave them. The good news is that humans have higher brain function that allows us to overcome our primal instincts. Ask anyone who has been on a healthy diet for 6 weeks or longer and they will tell you that their taste preferences have changed. They have come to prefer the full blend of flavors from fresh fruits and vegetables to the bland, sugary sweet foods they used to crave. They have come to appreciate a variety of herbs and spices in their cooking over the saltiness of the foods they used to crave. Finally, they have learned to appreciate lower fat foods. Many of their old favorites now seem greasy.

The bottom line is that our natural affinity for sugar, salt, and fat can be overcome by switching a variety of flavorful whole, unprocessed foods. Of course, the key word here is "unprocessed." This is where Big Food Inc tries to lure us away from healthy foods.

Now that we better understand where food myths come from, let's turn our attention to what I call "The Top 10 Food Myths."

Food Myth #1: Chocolate Craziness

Sometimes you come across news that just seems too good to be true. The headlines saying that you can lose weight just by eating chocolate are a perfect example. Your first reaction when you heard that was probably "Sure, when pigs fly!"

But, it's such an enticing idea – one might even say a deliciously enticing idea. And, in today's world enticing ideas like this quickly gain a life of their own. They quickly become food myths. Two popular books have been written on the subject. Chocolate diet plans are springing up right and left. A quick scan of the internet even revealed a website saying that by investing a mere $1,250 in a training course you could become a "Certified Chocolate Weight Loss Coach" earning $50,000/year. If you like chocolate as much as most people you are probably wondering if it could possibly be true.

The idea that chocolate could help you lose weight does have some support. There are three published clinical studies[20-22] suggesting that chocolate consumption is associated with lower weight. While that sounds impressive, they were all association studies. They looked at a cross section of the population and asked if chocolate intake was associated with BMI (a measure of obesity). You will remember that association studies have a couple of very important limitations:

- They are merely measuring associations. They don't prove cause and effect. Was it the chocolate that caused the lower weight, or was it something else that those populations were doing? We don't really know.

- They also don't tell us why an association occurs. In many ways, this is the old chicken and egg conundrum. Which comes first? In this case the question is whether the people in the studies became obese because they ate less chocolate – or did they eat less chocolate because they were obese and were trying to control their calories? Again, we have no way of knowing.

Chocolate is relatively rich in fat and high in calories. It's not your typical diet food. On the surface, it seems implausible that eating chocolate could help you lose weight. Scientists love to poke holes in implausible hypotheses, so it is no surprise that a recent study[23] has poked some huge holes in the "chocolate causes weight loss" hypothesis. This study analyzed data from over 12,000 participants in the Atherosclerosis Risk in Community (ARIC) Study. This was also an association study, but it was a prospective, association study. That's just a fancy scientific term which means that the study followed a cross section of the population over time, rather than just asking what that population group looked like at a single time point.

The authors of the study assessed frequency of chocolate intake and weight for every individual in the study at two separate times 6 years apart. The results were enlightening:

- When they looked at a cross section of the population at either time point, their results were the same as the previous three studies – namely those who consumed the most chocolate weighed less. So, the association data were consistent. Overweight people consume less chocolate. But, that still doesn't tell us why they consume less chocolate.

- However, when they followed individuals in the study over 6 years, those who consumed the most chocolate at the beginning of the study gained the most weight. The chocolate eaters were skinnier than the non-chocolate eaters at the beginning of the study, but they gained more weight as the study progressed. And, the more chocolate they consumed the more weight they gained over the next 6 years. [No surprise here. Calories still count.]

- When they specifically looked at the population who had developed an obesity-related illness between the first and second time point, they found that by the end of the study those participants had:
  - Decreased chocolate intake by 37%
  - Decreased fat intake by 4.5%
  - Increased fruit intake by 20%
  - Increased vegetable intake by 17%

In short, this study is more consistent with the "obesity causes reduced chocolate intake" model than the "reduced chocolate intake causes obesity" model. Simply put, if you are trying to lose weight, sweets like chocolate are probably among the first things to go. This is a perfect example of how clinical studies that just look at associations can give misleading results. The pigs were flying.

Food Myth #2: Sugar Silliness

Let's start with something that everyone agrees on. We consume way too much sugar in this country. The average American consumes 66 pounds of added sugar every year. That is up from 4 pounds of added sugar per year at the turn of the century. It translates into 23 teaspoons per day, much of it hidden in processed and convenience foods. In contrast, the American Heart Association recommends no more than 6 teaspoons per day for women and 9 teaspoons per day for men. That is less than you would find in a typical soda.

Once we go beyond agreeing that we are consuming too much sugar, it gets confusing. There are probably more myths around sugar than around any other food component. Each of these myths is based on a kernel of truth. However, before I debunk the sugar myths, let's start by looking at how we came to be eating so much sugar.

The Great Breakfast Cereal Debacle – How Did Our Diets Get So Bad?

It's hard to believe that breakfast cereals started as health food, but they did. Dr. John Harvey Kellogg was a Seventh-day Adventist who took over the Western Reform Health Institute in 1877 and renamed it the Battle Creek Sanitarium. It gained prominence as a health resort where people went to be healed through a combination of physical activity and healthy eating. Dr. Kellogg invented Corn Flakes in 1878 as a healthier alternative to the high-fat breakfasts most Americans were consuming at that time. Corn Flakes had less than 5% sugar. It was a great idea for its time, but what happened next is nothing short of appalling.

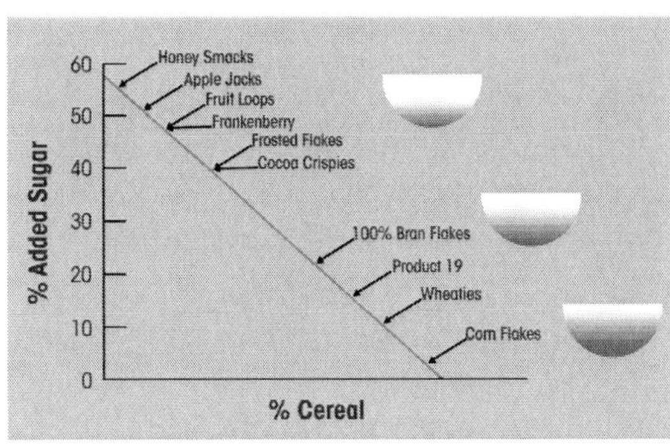

It is a perfect example of how Big Food Inc leads us astray. The graphic I have created illustrates what the major food companies have done to breakfast cereals over the decades since them. Other food companies soon brought out competing products. Cereals like Wheaties and Rice Krispies were still pretty healthy, but they had a bit more sugar, which gave them better consumer appeal. As soon as the food companies figured out that sugar increased their sales, the race was on. The percentage sugar increased to 40%, then to 50%, and now to almost 60%. No sane parent would fill their child's cereal bowl half full with sugar, but that is exactly what they are doing when they feed them some of today's breakfast cereals. The food companies are hiding the outrageous sugar content of their cereals with slogans like "Just a touch of honey." Speaking of deception, can anyone tell me how you label a product with 20% sugar 100% Bran Flakes?

A Rose By Any Other Name – Which Sugar Is Best?

There is a saying: "With age comes wisdom." However, I have observed that is not always the case. Let me paraphrase that saying as "With age comes perspective" and share some perspectives with you. When I was a young man back in the 60s and 70s, sugar-sweetened beverages primarily contained sucrose (table sugar) or glucose (also known as dextrose). Back then it was sucrose (table sugar) that was considered to be the root of all evil. Books like "Sugar Blues" popularized its villainy. We were told to avoid everything white – that would be table sugar, white flour and milk.

But sucrose was never the villain that it was said to be. Sucrose is a perfectly natural sugar and it is perfectly healthy in small amounts. The problem was that we were consuming way too much. That "teaspoon of sugar to help the medicine go down" had grown until sugar made up 10-15% of the calories in the American diet. In short, we had become addicted to sweetness.

Where was most of that sugar coming from? You guessed it – sodas, snack foods and processed foods. Of the 66 pounds/year of added sugar in the American diet, 37.1% comes from sugar-sweetened beverages, 19.8% comes from desserts, 8.9% comes from fruit drinks, and 5.8% comes from candy. In short, 71.6% of the added sugar we consume each year comes from sodas and junk food. The rest is hidden in the processed foods we eat.

The experts recommended that we cut back on all those processed foods and start eating more fresh fruits and vegetables. They are a bit less sweet, but so much healthier. But what did the American public do? We didn't want to give up the sweet stuff that we'd been accustomed to. More importantly, the food industry (Big Food Inc) didn't want us eating whole foods rather than the processed foods they were selling, so they obliged us by substituting fructose or high fructose corn syrup for sugar in all our favorite sodas, junk foods and processed foods.

What's wrong with that? After all, high fructose corn syrup contains a mixture of fructose and glucose. It is derived from corn. There is some processing required, but it meets the FDA's definition of natural. And, fructose is the major sugar found in many fruits, which are among the healthiest of foods. Even better, fructose does not produce the same spike in blood sugar that other sugars do.

However, in today's world, fructose and high fructose corn syrup are the sugars that are vilified. Some "experts" will tell you to avoid them at all costs. The "knock" on fructose and high fructose corn syrup is that they increase visceral fat (also known as belly fat), which increases the risk of insulin resistance, elevated triglycerides and type 2 diabetes – among other things. If that sounds familiar, it should. It is almost exactly what we were told about sucrose in the 60s and 70s.

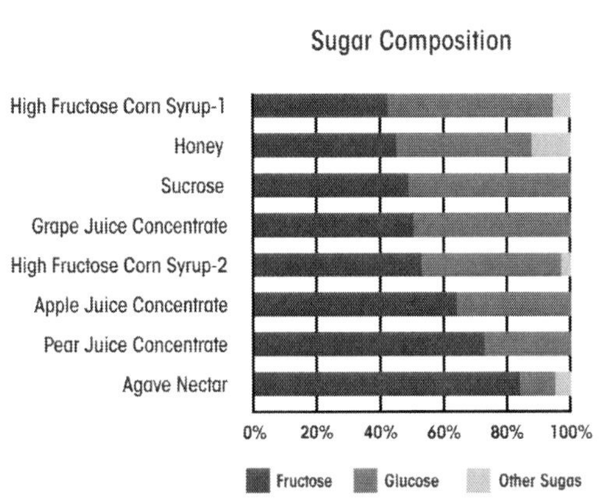

If we are to avoid foods sweetened with fructose and high fructose corn syrup, the question is: "What would you use in their place?" As the graphic I created illustrates, honey, molasses, maple syrup, or grape juice concentrate (used as natural sweeteners in a lot of "health" foods), table sugar (sucrose), raw sugar, evaporated cane juice and brown sugar all have an almost identical composition of fructose and glucose as does high fructose corn syrup. [Note: High fructose corn syrup comes in a variety of blends ranging from around 40% fructose to over 50% fructose depending on the food it will be used with. That is why you see high fructose corn syrup listed twice in the figure.] On the high end, apple and pear juice concentrates have more fructose than any high fructose corn syrup blend, and agave sugar is 85% fructose.

Clinical studies show that those similarities in sugar composition result in similar detrimental health consequences. For example, in one study[24] people consuming beverages sweetened with sucrose gained just as much belly fat as people consuming beverages sweetened with fructose. In other studies[25,26] people consuming large amounts of fruit juice had just as much risk of obesity and diabetes as those consuming large amounts of sodas.

The bottom line is that in the real world, there are no sugar heroes, and there are no sugar villains. If we were to consume 66 pounds of honey instead of 66 pounds of high fructose corn syrup per year, the health consequences would likely be almost the same. Of course, that will never happen. There just aren't enough bees. The same can be said for sucrose (the original sin) and for the sugar alcohols (sorbitol, mannitol, maltitol, erythritol, etc.) that are starting to find their way into a lot of processed foods.

The isn't in the sugar itself, it is in the amount that we are consuming and the foods in which we are consuming it. So, let's turn our attention to foods rather than sugars.

Is It The Sugar Or Is It The Food?

As I said at the beginning of the article, almost every expert agrees that Americans should cut down on the amount of sugar we are consuming. However, for some people this has become a "sugar phobia." They have sworn that "sugar shall never touch their lips." Not only do they avoid sugar-sweetened sodas and junk food, but they also have become avid label readers. They scour the label of every food they see and reject it if they find any form of sugar listed as an ingredient. Is this degree of sugar avoidance justified?

Let me add some perspective to the argument:

1) If you just take the studies at face value, sugar does, indeed, look villainous. Excess sugar consumption is associated with increased risk of obesity[27,28], diabetes[29], and heart disease[30,31]. However, when you look a little closer, you find that most of these studies have been done by looking at the correlation of each of these conditions with sugar-sweetened beverage consumption (sodas and fruit juices). The remaining few studies have looked at the correlation with total "added sugar" consumption, but you will remember that 71.6% of added sugar comes from sugar-sweetened beverages and junk food. None of the studies looked at the sugar from healthy foods like fruits, vegetables, and whole grains because there is ample evidence that those foods decrease the risk of obesity, diabetes, and heart disease.

2) If apples had a nutrition label, it would list 16 grams of sugar in a medium, 80-calorie apple, which corresponds to about 80% of the calories in that apple. The sugar in an apple is about the same proportion of fructose and glucose found in high fructose corn syrup. Apples are not unique. The nutrition label would read about the same on most other fruits. Does that mean you should avoid fruits? I think not.

The obvious question is: "Why are the same sugars, in about the same amounts, unhealthy in sodas and healthy in fruits?" Let's go back to those studies I just mentioned – the ones that are often used to vilify sugars. They are all association studies, the association of sugar intake with obesity and various diseases. You will remember the weakness of association studies is that the association could be with something else that is tightly correlated with the variable (sugar intake) you are measuring. Could it be the food that is the problem, not the sugar?

If we look at healthy foods (fruits, vegetables, whole grains) they are chock full of vitamins, minerals, phytonutrients, fiber, and (sometimes) protein. Fiber and protein slow the absorption of sugar into the bloodstream. Blood sugar levels rise slowly and are sustained at relatively low levels for a substantial length of time. In sodas there is nothing to slow the absorption of blood sugar. You get a rapid rise in blood sugar followed by an equally rapid fall. The same is true of junk foods consisting primarily of sugar, refined flour and/or fat.

Another consideration is something called caloric density. Here is a simple analogy I used to explain the concept of caloric density to medical students in my teaching days. There are about the same number of calories in a 2-ounce candy bar and a pound of apples (around 278 in the 2-ounce candy bar and 237 in a pound of apples). You can eat a 2-ounce candy bar and still be hungry. If you eat a pound of apples, you are done for a while. In this example, the 2-ounce candy bar had a high caloric density (a lot of calories in a small package). Perhaps a more familiar terminology would be the candy bar was just empty calories.

Putting all that together, you can start to understand why the foods the sugars are in are more important than the sugars themselves. When you consume sugars in the form of sugar-sweetened beverages or sugary junk foods, your appetite increases. We don't know for sure whether it is the intense sweetness of those foods, the increase and fall in blood sugar, or the high caloric density (lots of calories in a small package) that makes us hungrier. It doesn't matter. We crave more food, and it isn't usually fruits, vegetables, and complex carbohydrates we crave. It's more junk. That sets in motion a predictable sequence of events.

- We overeat. Those excess calories are stored as fat and we become obese.
- It's not just the fat you can see (belly fat) that is the problem. Some of that fat builds up in our liver and muscles. This sets up an unfortunate sequence of metabolic events.
    - The fat stores release inflammatory cytokines into our bloodstream. That causes inflammation. Inflammation increases the risk of many diseases including heart disease and cancer.
    - The fat stores also cause our cells to become resistant to insulin. That reduces the ability of our cells to take up glucose, which leads to hyperglycemia and type 2 diabetes.
    - Insulin resistance also causes the liver to overproduce cholesterol and triglycerides and pump them into the bloodstream. That increases the risk of heart disease.
    - Sugar-sweetened beverages and sugary junk foods also displace healthier foods from our diet. That leads to potential nutrient shortfalls that can increase our risk of many diseases.

However, none of this has to happen. The one thing that every successful weight loss program has in common is the elimination of sodas, junk foods, fast foods and convenience foods. Once you have eliminated those from your diet, you increase your chances of being at a healthy weight and being healthy long term.

Of course, the dilemma is what you, as an intrepid label reader, should do about protein supplements, meal replacement bars, or snack bars. They are supposed to be healthy, but the label lists one or more sugars. Even worse, the sugar content is higher than your favorite health guru recommends. In this case, a more useful concept is glycemic index, which is a measure of the effect of the food on your blood sugar levels. Healthy foods like apples may have a high sugar content, but they have a low glycemic index. The same may be true for the protein supplements and bars you are considering. Rather than looking at the sugar content, you should be looking for the term "low glycemic" on the label. That means there is enough fiber and protein in the food to slow the absorption of sugar into the bloodstream and stabilize your blood sugar levels.

Don't misunderstand me. I am not advocating for unlimited consumption of sugar. We should work on reducing the amount of sugar in our diet. On the other hand, we don't need to become so strict that we and our family end up to eating foods that taste like cardboard. We also don't want to replace natural sugars with artificial sweeteners. I will discuss the dangers of artificial sweeteners in the next section. In fact, we can go a long way toward reducing sugar just by eliminating sodas, junk foods, fast foods and convenience foods from our diet.

Summing It Up – Sugar Myths Debunked

Now you know there are no sugar heroes and no sugar villains. You know that it is the foods they are in, not the sugars themselves, that are important. You are fully armed to deflate some of the more pervasive sugar myths. Let's get started.

Sugar is a drug. We do have an instinctual desire for sugar, salt, and fat. That instinct served us well when they were scarce commodities, but does not serve us well today. Fortunately, we humans have a higher brain function. We can overcome our instincts.

Sugar "X" is bad. Substitute healthier sugars like "Y." (I used "X" and "Y" because "X" and "Y" have changed over the years. At present, "X" is high fructose corn syrup.) The bottom line is that there are no sugar heroes and no sugar villains. It is foods that are the problem.

Sugar is preferentially converted to fat and stored. In a healthy diet, most sugar is used for energy or stored as glycogen. Excess calories are stored as fat. It doesn't matter if those calories come from sugar, protein or fat. Furthermore, dietary fat requires no conversion. It can be stored "as is."

Sugar makes us fat. It is the sugar-sweetened beverages and sugary junk foods that make us fat. The same sugars in the same amounts in healthy foods do not make us fat.

Sugar causes diabetes. The idea that the spikes in blood sugar associated with sugar consumption wear out the pancreas is, and always has been, a myth. It is the excess fat stores associated with obesity that interfere with the insulin signaling pathway, which results in high blood sugar and type 2 diabetes. However, once you have diabetes, you need to limit sugar intake from sodas and sugary junk foods because high blood sugar is associated with diabetic complications. Sugar in healthy foods with a low glycemic index is not generally a problem for most diabetics.

Sugar causes inflammation. Excess fat stores associated with obesity are the primary cause of inflammation. Excess sugar makes no more contribution to those fat stores than excess protein or excess fat. However, high blood sugar due to diabetes or consumption of sodas and sugary junk foods also contributes to inflammation. Once again, sugar in healthy foods does not influence inflammation. For example, fruits are part of almost everyone's anti-inflammation diet.

Sugar causes heart disease, cancer, etc. Obesity and inflammation greatly increase the risk of these diseases. The studies suggesting a directly link between sugar consumption and those diseases looked at consumption of sugar-sweetened beverages and sugary junk foods, not healthy sugar-containing foods.

You should read labels and avoid any food containing more than a few grams of sugar. You don't need to restrict yourself to food products that taste like cardboard. However, you should read labels and you should avoid any sugar-containing processed food that doesn't say low glycemic on the label.

Food Myth #3: Diet Food Fantasy

Do Diet Sodas Help You Lose Weight?

Once Big Food Inc realized that Americans wanted to cut back on sugars, they were only too happy to oblige by creating a variety of artificial sweeteners and substituting them for sugar in beverages and a variety of junk and convenience foods. That should solve the problem, shouldn't it? That question might seem like a no-brainer. Eating calorie-free diet foods rather than sugar-sweetened foods with lots of calories must be helpful in keeping your weight under control. Right? Maybe not. Let's investigate that question by looking at calorie free diet sodas. What does the evidence actually show?

In 1960, 3.3% of Americans consumed diet sodas and 14% of us were obese. By 2010, 20% of us were consuming diet sodas and 41% of us were obese. It's clear that diet sodas aren't helping us solve the obesity epidemic, but are they actually part of the problem? Some recent studies suggest they might be.

For example, the San Antonio Heart Study[32] recorded consumption of diet sodas and regular sugar-sweetened sodas in 3,862 adults (average age 44) and measured the increase in BMI (a measure of obesity) over the next 7-8 years. That study found:

- Individuals consuming >21 diet sodas/week were almost two times more likely to become overweight or obese than individuals consuming no sodas.
- There was a clear dose response effect, with a 41% increased risk of becoming overweight or obese for each can or bottle of diet soda consumed/day.
- The increase in weight associated with diet soda consumption was just as great for those who were at normal weight at the beginning of the study as it was for those who were obese at the beginning of the study.
- Finally, in this study, the increase in weight associated with soda consumption was greater for diet sodas than it was for regular sodas.

Another major study[33] recorded diet and regular soda consumption in 6039 participants in the Framingham Heart Study (average age 53) and measured the increase in obesity (along with other parameters associated with metabolic syndrome or pre-diabetes) over the next 4 years. This study found:

- Individuals consuming one or more sodas/day had a 48% increased risk of becoming obese compared to people with infrequent soda consumption.
- In this study, the weight increase associated with soda consumption was virtually the same for diet sodas and regular sodas.

These and similar studies have been criticized because they are looking at associations, which, as you now know, do not prove cause and effect. For example, it's not always clear whether the people in those studies gained weight because they were consuming diet sodas or consuming diet sodas because they were overweight.

That argument is less persuasive for the San Antonio Heart Study, because the weight gain associated with diet soda consumption was also seen with people who were at normal weight at the beginning of the study. Still there is a need for good double-blind, placebo-controlled intervention studies.

There have been very few intervention studies in which one group of subjects were told to drink only diet sodas and the other group only regular sodas. Unfortunately, in those studies the total caloric intake of the diet soda group was also restricted. So, while the diet soda group did lose weight, it's not clear whether that weight loss was due to the diet sodas or the overall caloric restriction of the diet. Almost any diet will work if you have a dietitian looking over your shoulder and telling you how many calories to eat. However, in the real world we don't have dietitians telling us what to eat, and we appear to gain just as much weight with diet sodas as with sugar-sweetened sodas. "Why is that?" you might ask. Here are a couple of quotes I found particularly enlightening.

Dr. Barry Popkin, a colleague from the University of North Carolina, calls it the "Big Mac and Diet Coke" mentality. He says: "Especially in America, we have a lot of people who eat high-fat, high-sugar diets, but also drink diet sodas."

Why is that? Dr. David Katz from Yale University has research suggesting that artificial sweeteners may condition people to want to eat more sweet foods. He says: "Our taste buds don't really differentiate between sweet in sugar and sweet from, say, aspartame. The evidence that this sweet taste is addictive is pretty clear. What I have seen in my patients is that those who drink diet soda are more vulnerable to processed foods with added sugars."

Is that just coincidence or is something else going on here?

Some experts think that the effects are all psychological. The theory is that we think we are being virtuous by drinking zero calorie soft drinks, so we give ourselves permission to eat more high-sugar, high-fat, high-calorie foods.

Other experts think that the effects are physiological. One theory[34] is that artificial sweeteners activate an intestinal transporter that pumps dietary sugars into our bloodstream. This, in turn, causes blood sugar spikes that can lead to food cravings. Another theory[35] is that the high sweetness of both diet and regular soft drinks causes the brain to release chemicals that make us crave other sweet foods – so we eat more.

Even though the mechanism of the effect is unclear, the results are crystal clear. The authors of the Framingham Heart Study[33] concluded "In middle-aged adults, soft-drink consumption [both diet and regular] is associated with a higher prevalence of obesity and increased incidence of multiple metabolic risk factors [for diabetes and heart disease]."

So, the next time you reach for that diet soda or the packets of "zero calorie" sweeteners to add to your coffee or tea, just be aware that there is no good evidence that they are useful in helping you control your weight. And there is some evidence that they may even be making your weight control problems worse by encouraging you to eat high calorie foods to go along with them.

Are Diet Sodas Bad For You?

As you have just learned, it has become increasingly clear over the past few years that diet sodas are not the magic solution to weight control that everyone had hoped they will be. However, that's not the worst. Some studies are starting to suggest they may actually be bad for you.

For example, let's look at type 2 diabetes. There have been several clinical trials that have suggested that excess consumption of sugar-sweetened beverages may increase your risk of developing type 2 diabetes[29, 36]. Consequently, if you are at risk of developing type 2 diabetes, you've probably been advised by your doctor or dietitian to switch from sugar-sweetened beverages to artificially sweetened beverages or natural fruit juices. But, does that really work? Maybe not.

In fact, some studies have suggested that excess consumption of artificially sweetened beverages[37] or fruit juice[38] may be just as likely to lead to type 2 diabetes as consuming sugar-sweetened beverages. Once again, these studies were measuring associations, which do not prove cause and effect. Because of this limitation an international team of experts conducted a major systematic review and meta-analysis[39] of all reasonably well-designed prospective studies that measured the effect of beverage consumption on the development of type 2 diabetes over time. They evaluated the data from 17 studies that represented 38,253 people who developed type 2 diabetes over a period of at least two years. They used the most rigorous statistical analysis methods available, and they interpreted their results very cautiously. In short, this was a major study. So, what did the study show?

- An additional one serving per day of a sugar-sweetened beverage was associated with an 18% increase in your risk of developing type 2 diabetes. When you correct for obesity, the increased risk is 13%. (Note: We are talking about an 8-ounce serving here, not a 32-ounce Big Gulp or 64-ounce Double Gulp.)
- An additional one serving per day of an artificially-sweetened beverage was associated with a 25% increase in your risk of developing type 2 diabetes. When you correct for obesity, the increased risk is 8%. (Note: This means that even lean people consuming diet sodas daily for 2 years or more may have a slightly increased risk of developing type 2 diabetes.)

In short, if you want to decrease your risk of developing type 2 diabetes, neither sugar-sweetened nor diet sodas appear to be a particularly good choice.

The story with heart disease isn't any better. A recent study[40] followed roughly 2,500 New Yorkers over the age of 40 for 10 years. The study participants were divided into groups based on diet soda consumption: "none" (less than 1 per month), "light" (1 diet soda a month to 6 diet sodas a week), or "daily" (1 or more a day). After 10 years, the daily diet soda drinkers were more likely to have had a stroke or heart attack, or to have died from vascular disease. There was no increased risk of vascular events associated with regular soft drinks or light diet soft drink consumption. The increased risk for daily diet soda consumption remained even after controlling for smoking, exercise, weight, sodium intake, high cholesterol, and other factors that could have contributed to the difference.

Even more alarming is a recent study[41] suggesting that diet soda consumption may dramatically increase your risk of stroke. This study looked at 2888 participants of the Framingham Heart Study. The participants evaluated for risk of stroke had a mean age of 62 on enrollment. They were followed for 10 years. Three food frequency questionnaires were administered during that 10-year period to evaluate consumption of diet and sugar-sweetened sodas. The results of the study were:

- People consuming at least one diet soda per day over a 10-year period were 3X more likely to have a stroke than people consuming no diet sodas.
- When the data were corrected for hypertension, cardiovascular disease, and obesity (waist to hip ratio) diet sodas still increased the risk of having a stroke by 2.6-fold.

- No increased risk of stroke was seen for people consuming sugar-sweetened beverages. This is particularly concerning because it suggests switching from sugar-sweetened sodas to diet sodas may cause more harm than if people just continued drinking sugar-sweetened sodas.

These studies measure associations, not cause and effect. None of them is definitive by itself, but the evidence is starting to accumulate that diet sodas may not be a healthy choice.

What Do The Experts Say?

Many dietitians and doctors desperately want to believe that diet sodas and artificially sweetened foods are the solution to the global obesity epidemic because they have so few other viable options. Thus, the safety and efficacy of diet sodas remains a controversial issue. Recently, an international consortium of experts dedicated to solving the global obesity epidemic reviewed all the pertinent literature on diet sodas. They then published a position paper[42] on whether artificially sweetened beverages were of value in responding to the global obesity crisis.

These authors concluded:

- "In summary, the available evidence…does not consistently demonstrate that artificially-sweetened beverages are effective for weight loss or preventing metabolic abnormalities [pre-diabetes and diabetes]. Evidence on the impact of artificially-sweetened beverages on child health is even more limited and inconclusive than in adults."
- "The absence of evidence to support the role of artificially sweetened beverages in preventing weight gain and the lack of studies on their long-term effects on health strengthen the position that artificially-sweetened

> beverages should not be promoted as part of a healthy diet."

As you might expect these studies have caused quite a bit of controversy. Some experts have embraced these studies and have concluded that health professionals should stop recommending diet sodas as a safe and effective alternative to sugar-sweetened sodas. Others have been unwilling to change their recommendation of diet sodas for people who are obese and/or diabetic. Their rationale is threefold:

- These studies merely show that diet soda consumption is associated with weight gain, diabetes, heart disease, stroke and Alzheimer's. Association does not prove causation, so their viewpoint is that there is no conclusive proof that diet sodas cause weight gain and health risks.
- The obesity epidemic is a major health crisis, and consumption of sugar-sweetened beverages plays an important role in weight gain.
- They are convinced that most people are so addicted to the sweet taste of sugar that they would be unwilling to switch to calorie-free options like water or herbal teas.

In short, they are desperately clinging to the hope that substituting diet sodas for sugar-sweetened sodas will put a dent in the obesity crisis.

I side with the experts on global obesity who looked at all the available data and concluded there is no convincing evidence that diet sodas are either safe or effective. If the conversation were just centered around weight gain, diabetes, and heart disease, this could be considered an academic discussion. One could argue that diet sodas might have some benefit, and, at the worst, would have the same health risks as the regular sodas they replaced. However, the possibility that diet sodas may increase the risk of stroke is a game-changer in my mind. That's because consumption of sugar-sweetened sodas did not appear to increase the risk of stroke in that study. If true, that means substitution of diet sodas for sugar-sweetened sodas is not a neutral substitution. It could cause serious harm.

With no good evidence that diet sodas help people control weight and the possibility that they may have serious health risks, it is difficult to see how anyone in good conscience can continue to recommend diet sodas in place of regular sodas. My recommendation is to substitute water and other unsweetened beverages for the sugar-sweetened beverages you are currently consuming. If you crave the fizz of sodas, drink carbonated water. If you need more taste, try herbal teas or infuse water with slices of lemon, lime, or your favorite fruit.

Let me close by saying that I have focused this discussion on the efficacy and safety of diet sodas because there is a fair amount of experimental evidence that they are neither safe nor effective. These kinds of studies simply have not been done for any of the artificially sweetened junk and convenience "diet" foods that line the supermarket aisles. I suspect that when those studies are done, we will find out that "diet" foods are neither safe nor effective as well.

Food Myth #4: Saturated Fat Foolishness

The furor about saturated fats has to be one of the weirdest controversies in the nutrition world today. On one side you have the American Heart Association, the USDA, the Surgeon General's Office, the National Institutes of Health, and the top health experts in the country telling us that saturated fats are bad for us. We should minimize them in our diet. On the other side you have a ragtag group of doctors with popular websites telling us that carbohydrates are the problem. Saturated fats are good for us. We can eat as much as we want. It is the nutritional equivalent of fake news, but millions of Americans believe the myth that saturated fats are good for us. How can that be?

In part, it is because Americans love fats. We love fatty meats, butter, cheeses, and sour cream. They are part of our food heritage and culture. It is hard for us to believe the foods we grew up with might be bad for us. When someone tells us those foods are OK, we want to believe it. In part, it is also because we like to believe in conspiracies. We like to believe that those in a position of authority are hiding something. They are lying to us.

However, the biggest problem is that the science is confusing. It is very difficult to design really good studies about the health outcome of saturated fat consumption (more on that in a minute). As I mentioned earlier, one of the "secrets only scientists know" is that there will always be published studies on both sides of every issue. It is easy to "cherry pick" only the studies that support your viewpoint. With saturated fats, that is true in spades. There are dozens of studies you can pick on either side of the issue. Most of those studies have serious flaws, but the proponents of saturated fats are not trained scientists. They accept on face value every study that supports their viewpoint. And so, another myth is born.

Perhaps the best way to help you cut through the myths and help you make an informed decision on saturated fat is to share excerpts from two articles I have written on the subject. The first, "Are Saturated Fats Good For You?", was written in April 2014, soon after a meta-analysis was published claiming that saturated fats were good for you. The second, "Are Saturated Fats Bad For You?", was written in July 2017, shortly after the top heart experts in the country published a position paper on saturated fats for the American Heart Association.

Are Saturated Fats Good For You?

Bring out the fatted calf! Headlines are proclaiming that saturated fats don't increase your risk of heart disease – and that they may actually be good for you. The study[43] that attracted all the attention in the press was what we scientists call a meta-analysis. Basically, that is a study that combines the data from many clinical trials to improve the statistical power of the effect being studied. And it was a very large study. It included 81 clinical trials that looked at the effects of various types of fat on heart disease risk. Let's start by looking at the conclusions of the study. Then we will consider its validity.

When you read the study, you discover the headlines suggesting that saturated fats might be good for you were clearly misleading. The study concluded that saturated fats might not increase the risk of heart disease, but it never said that saturated fats were good for you. In short, the study concluded that:

- Saturated fats, monounsaturated fats and long chain omega-6 polyunsaturated fats did not affect heart disease risk.
- Long chain omega-3 polyunsaturated fats decreased heart disease risk.
- Trans fats increased heart disease risk.

If those conclusions are correct, they would represent a major paradigm shift. We have been told for years that we should limit saturated fats and replace them with unsaturated fats. Has that advice been wrong? Before we bring out the fatted calf and start heaping butter on our 12-ounce steaks, perhaps we should look at some of the limitations of this study. The first limitation is that we eat foods, not fats. Fortunately, the authors broke the data down into the effects of individual saturated fatty acids on heart disease risk. When you look at those data some interesting insights emerge. For example:

- Both palmitic acid and stearic acid, which are abundant in meats, increased the risk of heart disease.
- On the other hand, margaric acid, which is a minor saturated fatty in dairy foods, decreased the risk of heart disease.

So, while the net effect of saturated fats on heart disease risk may be zero, these data suggest:

- It is still a good idea to avoid fatty meats, especially red meats, if you want to reduce your risk of heart disease. When you focus on foods rather than fats, this fundamental advice has not changed in over 40 years!
- With fatty dairy foods, the situation is a little more uncertain. I'm not ready to tell you to break out the butter and whipped cream just yet, but recent research does suggest that dairy foods may have some beneficial effects that outweigh their saturated fat content.

Even more troubling, there was another weakness of this study, and it was a major one. The study did not ask what the individual clinical trials were replacing the saturated fats with. Many of them were simply replacing the saturated fats with carbohydrates. To understand why that is important, you have to go back to the research of Dr. Ancel Keys.

The whole concept of saturated fats increasing the risk of heart disease is based on the groundbreaking research of Dr. Ancel Keys in the 50s and 60s. But, it is important to understand what his research showed and didn't show. His research showed that when you replaced saturated fats with monounsaturated fats and/or polyunsaturated fats the risk of heart disease was significantly reduced. He was the very first advocate of what we now call the Mediterranean diet. (He lived to 101 and his wife lived to 97, so he must have been on to something.)

Unfortunately, his diet advice got corrupted by the food industry. The mantra became low-fat diets, where the saturated fat was replaced with carbohydrates – mostly simple sugars and refined flours. Since diets containing a lot of simple sugars and refined flours also increase the risk of heart disease, you completely offset the benefits of getting rid of the saturated fats. Just in case you think that is outdated dietary advice, Dr. Keys' recommendations were confirmed by a major meta-analysis published in 2009. That study[44] showed once again that replacing saturated fats with carbohydrates had no effect on heart disease risk, while replacing them with polyunsaturated fats significantly reduced risk.

So, you can put the fatted calf back out to pasture. The headlines telling you that saturated fats don't increase the risk of heart disease were overstated and misleading. Furthermore, the study upon which those headlines were based suffers from a major shortcoming that calls its conclusions into question. Finally, even if you accept its data at face value, it does not represent a paradigm shift. It simply reaffirms much of the current dietary advice about foods we should avoid.

Are Saturated Fats Bad For You?

The Saturated Fat Wars started heating up again three years later when the American Heart Association (AHA) released a Presidential Advisory statement[45] on the dangers of saturated fats. Critics immediately started trying to discredit the report. What is the truth?

A Presidential Advisory is the AHA's highest-level health advisory. It is meant to guide public health policy by government agencies such as the US Surgeon General's office, the USDA, and the CDC. However, the warnings about the dangers of saturated fat are very much like the warnings about the dangers of global warming. They have their believers and their deniers, and both sides passionately defend their positions. I understand the passion of saturated fat deniers. As I said earlier, foods high in saturated fat are an integral part of our heritage and our culture. It is only natural to want to believe those foods are good for us.

Because of this, I knew the AHA advisory would be controversial. After all, if someone is telling us we need to give up the foods we love, they better have darn good evidence to back up their recommendations. I knew my readers would want a scientifically accurate evaluation of the evidence, so I carefully analyzed the research studies the AHA presented in support of their recommendations. Here is what I found:

This report was put together by the top heart disease experts, both physicians and research scientists, in the country. They examined over 50 years of research studies. They also examined meta-analyses that combined the results of multiple research studies. In short, they examined the entire body of scientific evidence on diet and heart disease.

The AHA committee used very rigorous criteria in selecting the best studies for their analysis. They only included randomized clinical trials that:

- **Had actual cardiovascular end points – heart attack, stroke, and deaths due to heart disease**. Studies looking at things like LDL, HDL, particle size, inflammation, etc. only give you part of the picture. They may, or may not, accurately predict the risk of dying from heart disease.
- **Lasted two years or more**. The fats we eat determine the fat composition of our cell membranes, and that is what ultimately determines our risk of dying from heart disease. However, changing the fat composition of our cell membranes does not occur overnight. It takes 2 years or more to achieve a 60-70% change in the fat composition of cell membranes. It also takes time for any intervention to meaningfully impact heart disease risk. Even with statin drugs, it takes 1-2 years before there

is a significant reduction in heart disease risk. Thus, studies of less than 2 years duration are doomed to fail.

- **Showed the subjects stuck with the new diet for the duration of the study**. Subjects often find it difficult to adhere long term to a diet to which they are not accustomed and revert to their more familiar diet. To show that subjects stuck to their diet requires either very close monitoring of what the subjects were eating or measurement of fat membrane composition to verify diet adherence, or both. Studies that only measured what the subjects were eating at the beginning of the study and then looked at outcomes months or years later may or may not be valid. Without any measurement of diet adherence, it is impossible to know.
- **Carefully controlled or measured what the saturated fats were replaced with**. The importance of this criterion will be clear when we look at the results of their study.

They then did a meta-analysis of what they referred to as "core randomized trials" that met all 4 criteria. In short, this was a very rigorous and well-done analysis.

The main findings of the report were:

- Replacing saturated fats from animal products with polyunsaturated fats from vegetable oils decreased the risk of heart disease by 29%.
    - o This is equivalent to statin therapy, without the side effects.
    - o The conclusions of this report applied equally to the saturated fats that come from meats and dairy products.
    - o Only 50% of the risk reduction came from lowering LDL cholesterol. The rest came from reduced

arterial inflammation, increased flexibility of the arteries, increased membrane fluidity and other factors.

- When the replacement of saturated fats with polyunsaturated fats occurred in the context of a heart-healthy diet such as the Mediterranean diet, heart disease risk was reduced by 47%.

What the saturated fats are replaced with is critically important. The authors of this report calculated what would happen if we were to replace just half of our saturated fat calories with equivalent calories from other foods. Replacing half of our saturated fat intake with:

- Polyunsaturated fats (vegetable oils and fish oil) lowers heart disease risk by 25%.
- Monounsaturated fats (olive oil and peanut oil) lowers heart disease risk by 15%.
- Complex carbohydrates (whole grains, fruits and vegetables) lowers heart disease risk by 9%.
- Refined carbohydrates and sugars (the kind of carbohydrates in the typical American Diet) slightly increases heart disease risk.
- Trans fats increases heart disease risk by 5%.

The saturated fat deniers have wasted no time trying to discredit the American Heart Association advisory. Maybe they can't bear the thought of having to give up their favorite fatty foods. Or maybe they just can't bear to admit they were wrong. However, their claims just don't hold water. Let me give you examples of some of their more outrageous claims.

- **The AHA (American Heart Association) is a tool of the pharmaceutical industry**. If the AHA were a tool of the pharmaceutical industry, I hardly think their report would have stated that replacing saturated fats with polyunsaturated fats was as effective as statin drugs at reducing heart attack risk.
- **The AHA is a tool of the food industry**. If the AHA were a tool of the food industry, I hardly think they would have recommended replacing fats from meat and dairy with polyunsaturated fats.
- **The AHA advisory was based on associations, which do not show cause and effect**. False. The AHA committee based their recommendations on randomized clinical trials, the strongest kind of evidence.
- **The AHA advisory was based on LDL cholesterol, which is an imperfect predictor of cardiovascular risk**. False. Again, the AHA committee based their recommendations on randomized clinical trials of cardiovascular outcomes, not on LDL levels.
- **The AHA committee ignored an early study in which replacing butter with polyunsaturated fats increased cardiovascular risk**. False. That study actually replaced butter with margarine. It was the first study showing that trans fats are worse for us than saturated fats.
- **The AHA committee ignored recent studies that did not fit their hypothesis**. False. They developed a valid set of scientific criteria for evaluating clinical studies. They simply eliminated those studies whose designs were faulty and did not permit a definitive conclusion.
- **The AHA recommends low-fat diets containing refined carbohydrates and sugary foods, which are even worse**. False. The AHA has consistently recommended low-fat diets with polyunsaturated fats and complex

> carbohydrates (whole grains, fruits and vegetables). It is the food industry that corrupted their message. More to the point, this AHA Presidential Advisory specifically recommended lowering saturated fats in the context of a heart-healthy diet like the Mediterranean diet.

In short, the saturated fat deniers have no persuasive counter-argument. The evidence that saturated fat causes heart disease is simply overwhelming. The time for debate is over. It should be obvious to any reasonable person that saturated fats increase our risk of heart disease. It should also be obvious that any diet claiming saturated fats are heart-healthy is a myth. There are no long-term studies to back up that claim.

It is time to consider what it would mean if everyone in this country were to follow the AHA recommendations and replace half of the saturated fat in our diet with polyunsaturated fat in the context of a heart-healthy diet like the Mediterranean diet. That would decrease our risk of heart disease by 47%.

- 800,000 Americans die of heart disease each year. 376,000 lives could be saved.
- Heart disease costs our nation $316 billion each year. $146 billion in health care dollars could be saved.
- Heart disease costs are expected to exceed $1 trillion by 2035. $470 billion in health care dollars could be saved.

Each of us can save our health and our lives by what we put into our mouths every day. In addition, our health care system will soon become financially non-viable if we continue to focus on disease treatment rather than prevention. Each of us can also save our health care system by what we put into our mouths every day.

Food Myth #5: Coconut Confusion

Coconut oil is a saturated fat, but lately we are being told that it is good for us. In fact, it is the latest miracle food. Bloggers and talk show hosts are telling us how healthy it is. We are being told to cook with it, spread it on our toast, and put it in our smoothies. We are told to be creative. The more coconut oil you can get into your diet, the better.

The hype is working. 72% of the American public now believes coconut oil is healthy. This is one of the reasons why the recent American Heart Association Presidential Advisory[45] on saturated fats has proven so controversial. Interestingly, most of the AHA advisory was about the linkage between saturated fats from meat and dairy and heart disease risk. Only one paragraph of the 24-page report was devoted to coconut oil, but the AHA recommendation to avoid coconut oil generated the lion's share of headlines.

Is Coconut Oil Bad For You?

The AHA advisory concluded that saturated fats from meat and dairy foods increased the risk of heart disease. This conclusion was based on randomized clinical trials in which the diet was carefully controlled for a period of at least two years.

In contrast to the saturated fats in meat and dairy, there have been no studies looking at the effect of coconut oil on cardiovascular outcomes. Instead, the authors of the AHA report relied on studies measuring the effect of coconut oil on LDL cholesterol levels. There have been 7 controlled trials in which coconut oil was compared with monounsaturated or polyunsaturated oils.

- Coconut oil raised LDL cholesterol in all 7 studies.
- The increase in LDL cholesterol in these studies was identical to that seen with butter, beef fat, or palm oil.

This evidence makes it probable that coconut oil increases the risk of heart disease. However, LDL is not a perfect predictor of heart disease risk. The only way to definitively prove that coconut oil increases the risk of heart disease would be to conduct clinical studies in which:

- Coconut oil was substituted for other fats in the diet.
- All other dietary components were kept the same.
- The study lasted at least 2 years.
- Adherence to the "coconut oil diet" was monitored.
- Cardiovascular outcomes were measured (heart attack, stroke, death from heart disease).

In short, one would need the same type of study that supports the AHA warning about saturated fats from meats and dairy. In the absence of this kind of study, there is no "smoking gun." We cannot definitively say that coconut oil increases the risk of heart disease.

Is Coconut Oil Healthy?

Does that mean all those people who have been claiming coconut oil is a health food are right? Probably not. At the very least, their health claims are grossly overstated.

Let's start with the obvious. In the absence of any long-term studies on the effect of coconut oil on cardiovascular outcomes, nobody can claim that coconut oil is heart-healthy. It might be, but it might also be just as bad for you as the saturated fats from meat and dairy. Its effect on LDL cholesterol suggests it might increase your risk of heart disease, but we simply do not know for certain.

I taught human metabolism to medical students for 40 years. I was also a research scientist who published in peer reviewed journals. When I look at the health claims for coconut oil on the internet, I am dismayed. Many of the claims are complete nonsense. Others sound plausible, but are based on an incomplete understanding of human metabolism. None of them would pass peer review, but, of course, there is no peer review on the internet.

In addition, some of the claims have been "cherry picked" from the literature. For example, claims that coconut oil increases metabolic rate or aids weight loss are based on short-term studies and ignore long-term studies showing those effects disappear over time. Let me review some of the more plausible-sounding claims for coconut oil.

Coconut oil increases HDL levels, which is heart-healthy. The effects of HDL cholesterol are complex. Elevated HDL levels are not always heart protective.

For example, a few years ago a pharmaceutical company developed a drug that raised HDL levels. They thought they had a blockbuster drug. You didn't need to exercise. You didn't need to lose weight. You would just pop their pill and your HDL levels would go up. There was only one problem. When they did the clinical studies, their drug had no effect on heart disease risk. It turns out it was exercise and weight loss that reduced heart disease risk, not the increase in HDL associated with exercise and weight loss.

The implications are profound. Just because something increases HDL levels does not mean it will reduce cardiovascular risk. You have to actually measure cardiovascular risk before claiming something is heart-healthy. That has not been done for coconut oil, so no one can claim it is heart-healthy.

Coconut oil consists of medium chain triglycerides, which are absorbed more readily than other fats. That is true, but it is of interest to you only if you suffer from a fat malabsorption disease. Otherwise, it is of little importance to you.

You will lose weight because the medium chain triglycerides in coconut oil are preferentially transported to the liver,

where the fats in coconut oil are converted to energy or released as ketones rather than being stored as fat. This is partially true, but it is misleading for three reasons.

- First, the fat in coconut oil actually has three possible fates in the liver. Some of it will be converted to energy, but only enough to meet the immediate energy needs of the liver. If carbohydrates are limited, the excess will be converted to ketones and exported to other tissues as an energy source. If carbohydrates are plentiful, the excess will be converted to long chain saturated fats identical to those found in meat and dairy and exported to other tissues for storage.
- Secondly, the maximal amount of ketones you can excrete in a day is 100 calories or less. In short, the calories from coconut oil aren't going anywhere. They will either be used as energy or stored as fat.
- Finally, nobody has repealed the laws of thermodynamics. If the fat in coconut oil is being used as an energy source by the liver and other tissues in your body, you need to ask what happens to the calories from the other components in your diet. If you are eating a typical American diet, the carbohydrates that would have been used for energy will be converted to fat and stored. If you are eating a low-carbohydrate diet, the other fats that would have been used for energy will simply be stored. Simply put, if you are preferentially using the calories from coconut oil for energy, the calories from the other foods in your diet don't just evaporate. They are stored as fat.

Coconut oil increases metabolic rate, which will help you lose weight. When you look at the studies, this is only a temporary effect. This is probably due to a phenomenon called "metabolic adaptation" that is often seen when one makes a dramatic shift in diet composition. Initially, you may see an increase in metabolic rate and weight loss. After a few weeks, the body adapts to the new diet, and your metabolic rate returns to normal.

Coconut oil is metabolized to ketones which have many beneficial effects. There is some truth to this claim, but not nearly as much as proponents claim. Furthermore, the amount of ketones produced by coconut oil will depend on the availability of carbohydrates. Much of the coconut oil in the context of a very low-carbohydrate diet will likely be converted to ketones. Coconut oil spread on a piece of bread or used in baking is more likely going to be converted to fat.

I could go on, but you get the point. The hype about the benefits of coconut oil sounds good, but is misleading. There may be some benefits, but in the absence of long-term studies we have no convincing evidence that coconut oil is good for us.

What Does This Mean For You?

When you started reading this section, you were probably hoping that I would settle the coconut oil controversy. Perhaps you were hoping that I would tell you the American Heart Association was right, and you should avoid coconut oil completely. More likely you were hoping I would tell you the coconut oil proponents were right, and you could continue looking for more ways to incorporate coconut oil into your diet. As usual, the truth is somewhere in between.

Coconut oil may increase our heart disease risk, but the evidence is not definitive. We cannot say with certainty that coconut oil is bad for us. On the other hand, most of the hype about the benefits of coconut oil is inaccurate or misleading. We have no well-designed, long-term studies on health outcomes from coconut oil use. We cannot say with certainty that coconut oil is good for us.

I recommend moderation. Small amounts of coconut oil are probably all right. If you have a particular recipe for which coconut oil gives the perfect flavor, go ahead and use it. Just don't add it to everything you eat.

More to the point, there are other oils we know to be healthy that you can use in place of coconut oil. If you are looking for monounsaturated oils, olive oil and avocado oil are your best bets. Olive oil can be used in salads and low temperature cooking. Avocado oil is better for high temperature cooking. Also, less frequently mentioned, safflower and sunflower oils are also good sources of monounsaturated fats.

If you are looking for a mixture of monounsaturated and polyunsaturated fats, safflower oil, canola oil and peanut oil are your best bets. Peanut oil is also good for high temperature cooking. Corn oil and soybean oil are your best sources of omega-6 polyunsaturated fats, while flaxseed oil is your best vegetable source of omega-3 polyunsaturated fats.

Food Myth #6: Protein Proficiency

One of the recurring nutrition controversies centers around how much protein Americans are getting. Some experts say that we are consuming too much protein, and that can lead to serious health issues. Other experts say that many of us may not be getting enough protein and those protein deficits can lead to problems. Once again, the truth is somewhere in between those extremes.

Are You Getting Too Much Protein?

The whole controversy was brought to a head by a recent article in the New York Times titled "Can You Get Too Much Protein?" The article appeared in late 2016 and received a lot of press. The New York Times asserted that most Americans were getting too much protein in their diet. They went on to imply that protein supplements were useless at best and might be downright harmful at worst.

If you happened to read that article, you were probably wondering whether it was true or just another example of media bias. However, the problem goes way beyond media bias. In today's online world everyone is a writer, and everyone is an editor. More importantly, news is instant. Newspapers and journalists no longer have the time and resources to fully research a topic before they publish it. When a story comes along that fits their bias, the temptation is strong to publish it immediately. The New York Times got some things right and other things wrong, so let me give you a more balanced perspective.

What Did The New York Times Get Right?

The New York Times didn't completely miss the mark. Here are a few things that they got right:

- Most Americans are getting more than the RDA for protein in their daily diets. They imply that is too much. However, the prevailing view among many nutrition experts today is that the RDA is too low for some groups, and many Americans are getting too little protein, not too much.
- They do acknowledge that there are groups who aren't getting enough protein, for example teenage girls, pregnant and lactating women, people over 60, and professional athletes. I would add, based on recent studies, that any adult who is engaged in a weight loss program and/or regular, vigorous workouts will also benefit from extra protein, especially after their workout. If you combine all those categories, we are talking about the majority of Americans not getting enough protein. The only exception is the otherwise healthy adults who are "couch potatoes."

- They are correct in saying that the average "couch potato" adult in the US doesn't need more protein. However, even the "couch potatoes" among us would benefit from more vegetable protein in place of some of the high-fat, high-cholesterol animal protein they are eating. They don't need more protein. They just need better protein.
- Finally, they are correct in saying many protein supplements are either unsafe or suffer from poor quality control. My advice is simple. Avoid those protein supplements making extravagant claims about "exploding" your muscles and giving you boundless energy. Also, choose protein supplements made by reputable companies that employ rigorous quality controls.

What Did The New York Times Get Wrong?

The main theme of their article was that most Americans were getting too much protein. They acknowledged that some nutritionists advocated consuming more protein but implied that most experts did not agree. That paradigm is 20 years old. The evidence has shifted. Most experts today feel that many Americans aren't getting enough protein. I will give some examples in the pages to follow.

They warned that high protein intake could be harmful. It could lead to increased risk of cancer, heart disease, diabetes and kidney disease. Let's put those claims into perspective.

- Increased risk of cancer is linked to high intake of animal protein, especially red meat and processed meats (more about that later). There is no evidence that vegetable protein increases your risk of cancer.
- Increased risk of heart disease and diabetes is linked to high intake of fat and cholesterol-rich animal proteins. Once again, there is no evidence that vegetable protein increases the risk of either heart disease or diabetes.

- In short, for these diseases it's the kind of protein, not the amount, that is the problem.
- As for kidney disease, it is clear that protein intake should be restricted when you have kidney disease. It is not clear that high protein intake can cause kidney disease in healthy adults.

As for protein supplements, they assumed that most people who used plant-based protein supplements just added them to the protein they were already eating. If that were true, it might be a problem. However, most people use plant-based protein supplements in place of some of the high-fat animal protein in their diet. They aren't necessarily eating more protein. They are eating healthier protein.

What Do Recent Studies Show?

If we look at recent publications on the subject, it is clear the New York Times article did not accurately report what current studies show about the protein needs of Americans. Here are just a few examples:

High-protein diets improve physical function and weight loss in older adults. In this study[46] participants on the high-protein diet:

- Lost 15% more weight than those on the low-protein diet. More importantly, the high-protein group had:
    - 60% better retention of lean body mass (muscle).
    - 25% better loss of fat mass.
- They also performed substantially better on physical function tests than the low-protein group. There was no exercise component to this study. The improvement in physical function was solely related to the better

retention of muscle mass and the greater loss of fat mass in the high-protein group.

High-protein diets improve fat mass loss and muscle mass gain in young adults on a weight loss diet. In this study[47] the high-protein group:

- Had 33% greater loss of fat mass than the low-protein group.
- Increased muscle mass by an average of 2.6 pounds compared to no change in the low-protein group.

High-protein diets improve satiety. In this study[48] the high-protein group:

- Reported greater satiety and less hunger between breakfast and lunch.
- Consumed 12% fewer calories at lunch.

These are just a few recent studies. There are dozens of other studies that come to the same conclusions. The increased protein needs of teenage girls and pregnant and lactating women have been recognized for years. However, the increased protein needs of people over 60, dieters, and athletes is new science, so I will investigate the evidence with you in a bit more detail.

Protein Needs Of Older Adults

Many Americans suffer from sarcopenia (loss of muscle mass) as they age. Starting at age 50 we lose 1-2% of muscle mass and 1.5% of muscle strength each year. Over age 65 this increases to 3% loss of strength/year. That's a 30% loss by age 75 and a 60% loss by age 85! Some of you may be saying "So what? I wasn't planning on being a champion weightlifter in my golden years." The "So what" is that loss of muscle mass leads to loss of mobility, a tendency to fall (which often leads to debilitating bone fractures) and a lower metabolic rate – which leads to obesity and all the illnesses that go along with obesity.

Fortunately, sarcopenia is not an inevitable consequence of aging. There are things that we can do to prevent it. The most important thing that we can do to prevent muscle loss as we age is to exercise – and I'm talking about resistance (weight) training, not just aerobic exercise. But we also need to look at our protein intake and the leucine content of the protein we eat. Protein is important because our muscle fibers are made of protein. Leucine is an essential amino acid. It is also important because it stimulates the muscle's ability to make new protein.

Our Protein Needs Increase As We Age

Interestingly, our protein needs actually increase as we age. For example, Campbell et al[49] showed several years ago that RDA levels of protein were not sufficient to maintain muscle mass in either men or women aged 55 to 77 years old.

The RDA for protein is currently set at 0.8 g of protein/kg of body weight/day for all adults (56 grams of protein/day for men and 46 grams of protein/day for women). However, an international team of experts recently recommended setting the protein allowance at 1.0 to 1.2 grams of protein/kg of body weight/day for adults over 65. That would correspond to 70-84 grams/day for men over 65 and 58-69 grams/day for women over 65.

Dr. Jose Antonio, head of the International Society of Sports Nutrition, recently said, "It is about time that clinicians realized that consuming protein above the RDA is needed to ameliorate the loss of muscle protein with age. Adhering to the RDA for protein would be like whitewater rafting without a paddle. It's just plain dumb."

Protein Intake Should Be Spread Throughout The Day

When we consume the protein is also important. Forget that continental breakfast, salad for lunch and protein-rich dinner. As we age we increasingly need high-quality protein at every meal.

In one study[50], young adults (average age = 31) experienced increased muscle protein synthesis when they consumed as little as 15 grams of protein at a meal, but older adults (average age = 68) experienced no increase in muscle protein synthesis in response to the same low-protein meal. However, when the amount of protein in a meal was increased to 30 grams (equivalent to a 4-oz piece of chicken or beef) both younger and older adults were able to use that protein to build muscle[51].

But, 30 grams seems to be about optimal. Protein intakes above 30 grams in a single meal resulted in no further increase in muscle protein synthesis[52], which means you can't hope to get all the muscle-building benefits of protein in a single meal. Because of these studies most experts recommend that we "golden agers" aim for 20 to 30 grams of high-quality protein with every meal.

How Much Leucine Do We Need?

The story with leucine is similar. 1.7 grams of leucine following exercise was sufficient to increase muscle mass for younger adults. However, 2.7 grams was needed to increase muscle protein synthesis following exercise in older adults[53]. So, the experts recommend that older adults get 2.5-3 grams of leucine in the protein we consume following workouts to maximize the effect of the workout on increasing muscle mass.

Where Do We Get The Protein And Leucine We Need?

So, where do we get the amount of protein and leucine that we are looking for? If you want to get them from food alone,

4-oz servings of meat are a good starting place – with chicken being the best (35 grams of protein and 2.7 grams of leucine). Dairy, eggs and vegetable foods are much lower in leucine, protein or both.

Unfortunately, I keep running into seniors who are fully convinced that broccoli and tofu will meet their protein needs. I fully understand the rationale for choosing vegetarian protein sources, but you need a bit more than broccoli and tofu if you are going to meet your protein needs in your golden years. For example, a 4-ounce serving of tofu provides only 10 grams of protein and 0.8 grams of leucine, and a 1-cup serving of broccoli provides only 4.2 grams of protein and a miserly 0.36 grams of leucine. That makes it very difficult to meet your target of 20-30 grams of protein and 2.5-3 grams of leucine with each meal.

I'm not saying that you can't get enough protein and leucine to maintain muscle mass on a vegetarian diet. However, you will need to focus on high-protein vegetable foods. Among vegetable foods, soybeans are the winner with 30 grams of protein and 2.3 grams of leucine in a 1-cup serving. Most other beans and legumes provide 15-16 grams of protein and 1.2-1.3 of leucine per serving. Because they are higher in calories, we usually consider 1 ounce as a serving size for nuts and seeds. That generally provides 5-7 grams of protein and 0.4-0.5 grams of leucine. With a little advanced planning you should have no trouble meeting your protein and leucine needs. However, if advanced planning is not your forte, you can also use plant-based protein supplements with added leucine to help meet your protein and leucine targets.

Protein And Weight Loss

Now let's turn our attention the question of optimal protein intake when you are trying to lose weight. There are lots of diets out there – high-fat, low-carb, Paleolithic, blood type, exotic juices, magic pills and potions. But recently, high-protein diets are also getting a lot of press. That is because they preserve muscle mass and preferentially decrease fat mass. That is huge because:

- It's the fat – not the pounds – that causes most of the health problems.
- Muscle burns more calories than fat, so preserving muscle mass helps keep your metabolic rate high without dangerous herbs or stimulants – and keeping your metabolic rate high helps prevent both the plateau and yo-yo (weight regain) characteristic of so many diets.
- When you lose fat and retain muscle, you are reshaping your body – and that's why most people are dieting to begin with.

The groundbreaking research in this area was done by Dr. Donald K Layman and colleagues at the University of Illinois. They have published seven clinical studies comparing the efficacy of isocaloric high-protein diets (40% carbohydrate, 30% protein, 30% fat) containing 10 g of leucine (total for the day), and traditional low-fat, high-carbohydrate diets (55% carbohydrate, 15% protein, 30% fat) containing 2 g of leucine. They have enrolled a total of 421 adults (age ~50, BMI ~33) in these studies. The duration of the studies ranged from 10 weeks[54] to 4 months[55,56] to 1 year[57].

Their studies have consistently shown that:

- The high-protein, high-leucine diet promoted retention of muscle mass and preferential loss of fat mass compared to the high-carbohydrate, low-fat diet.
- The high-protein, high-leucine diet gave greater satiety, which resulted in better long-term retention of weight loss than the high-carbohydrate, low-fat diet.

- The high-protein, high-leucine diet gave improved insulin sensitivity (as measured by glycemic and insulin response to a test meal) compared to the high-carbohydrate, low-fat diet.
- The high-protein, high-leucine diet gave a greater reduction in triglyceride levels and a greater reduction in the triglyceride/HDL ratio than the high-carbohydrate diet.
- Exercise also promoted retention of muscle mass and loss of fat mass, and the effects of exercise and the high-protein, high-leucine diet were additive.
- The weight loss and changes in body composition (muscle retention and fat loss) were retained during an 8-month maintenance phase[58].
- The diet worked equally well in overweight, elderly women[59].
- The diet worked best when the protein was spread out evenly during the day rather than being concentrated in the evening meal[60].

In short, these studies have shown that the high-protein, high-leucine diets offer all the advantages of low-carbohydrate diets (improved insulin sensitivity, low triglyceride levels) without reliance on high levels of unhealthy fats in the diet. Furthermore, the high-protein, high-leucine diets provide the additional advantage of preserving muscle mass and promoting greater loss of fat mass.

Their research has been confirmed by dozens of studies by independent investigators at other universities. One recent study is of interest because it has helped define how much protein is optimal for muscle mass retention and fat loss during caloric restriction. This was a randomized control study with[61] healthy young men and women who were only borderline overweight (BMI = 25). These volunteers were put on a 21-day weight loss program in which calories were reduced by 30% and exercise was increased by 10%. They were divided into 3 groups:

- One group was assigned a diet containing the RDA for protein (about 14% of calories in this study design).
- The second group's diet contained 2X the RDA for protein (28% of calories).
- The third group's diet contained 3X the RDA for protein (42% of calories).

In the RDA protein group carbohydrates were 56% of calories, and fat was 30% of calories. In the other two groups, the carbohydrate and fat content of the diets was decreased proportionally. In other words, the diet was neither low-carb or low-fat.

The results were as follows:

- Weight loss (7 pounds in 21 days) was the same on all 3 diets.
- The high-protein (28% and 42%) diets caused almost 2X more fat loss (5 pounds versus 2.8 pounds) than the diet supplying the RDA amount of protein.
- The high-protein (28% and 42%) diets caused 2X less muscle loss (2.1 pounds versus 4.2 pounds) than the diet supplying the RDA amount of protein.
- In case you didn't notice, there was no difference in overall results between the 28% (2X the RDA) and 42% (3X the RDA) diets. This clearly sets an upper limit on how much protein is needed to preserve muscle mass during weight loss.

There are two important implications of these studies:

#1: Preferential fat loss is the "Holy Grail" of the diet world. However, it is hard to deliver on that promise. When you reduce calories, the body's natural response is to burn both fat and protein for energy. Many diets claim preferential fat loss, but don't deliver. Other diets use dangerous stimulants to achieve preferential fat loss. These studies show you can achieve preferential fat loss with foods alone if your protein intake is high enough.

#2: Low-carb diets often contain unhealthy fats. Low-fat diets often contain unhealthy carbs. Dr. Layman's diet is low-fat, but, more importantly, it is designed with healthy fats and healthy carbohydrates. You don't need to follow an unhealthy diet to lose weight.

Protein Needs Of Athletes

There is lots of conflicting information about how much protein athletes should be getting. Some experts say athletes need more protein. Others say they get plenty of protein in the standard American diet. Because of all the conflicting advice, I thought it would be worthwhile to share with you the International Society of Sports Nutrition's (ISSN) recently published Position Statement[62] on protein and exercise. It represents the consensus position of the world's top exercise physiologists, sports nutritionists, and coaches.

Before summarizing the International Society of Sports Nutrition (ISSN) recommendations, I should start by pointing out that these recommendations are focused on the effect of protein on exercise performance. They are also focused more on high-performance athletes than on those of us who are just trying to stay fit. Here are the ISSN recommendations with my comments:

#1: "An acute exercise stimulus, particularly resistance exercise, and protein ingestion both stimulate muscle protein synthesis and are synergistic." In simple English, exercise and protein work synergistically to help you increase muscle mass.

#2: "For building and maintaining muscle mass... an overall daily protein intake in the range of 0.6-0.9 gm/pound body weight/day is sufficient for most exercising individuals." This is 1.7-2.5 times the RDA for sedentary individuals, and is more appropriate for elite athletes than for your average weekend warrior or fitness enthusiast.

They make the point that protein alone is sufficient for increasing muscle mass following resistance training. However, I prefer some carbohydrates with a protein meal or supplement because of a phenomenon called "protein sparing." In the absence of carbohydrates, some of the ingested protein is converted to glucose to restore blood glucose levels and muscle glycogen stores. If you include carbohydrates with the protein, the carbohydrates will be used to restore blood glucose and glycogen, and all the protein can be used to increase muscle mass.

#3: "There is novel evidence that suggests higher protein intake (>1.36 gm/pound body weight/day) may promote loss of fat mass in resistance-trained individuals." This recommendation is primarily for bodybuilders.

#4: "Optimal protein intake per serving...depends on age and [the intensity of] recent resistance exercise. General recommendations are...a dose of 20-40g." With respect to intensity of exercise, most of us engage in moderate intensity exercise and should aim for 20-30g. As I pointed out earlier, young people require less protein following exercise (~20 g) than older people (~30g). Higher doses are more appropriate for elite athletes engaged in high-intensity training.

#5: "Acute protein doses should strive to contain 700-3,000 mg of leucine...in addition to a balanced array of the essential amino acids." As I pointed out earlier, older people also need more leucine (2,500-3,000 mg) than younger people (700-1,700 mg). It is also worth noting that in their position statement, the ISSN did not recommend any of the other ingredients that you often find in those "Mega Muscle" protein supplements.

#6: "These protein doses should be evenly distributed, every 3-4 h, across the day." If you consume too much protein at one time, the excess will not be used for building muscle. It will be used for building fat stores.

#7: "The optimal time period during which to ingest protein is likely a matter of individual tolerance…However, the anabolic effect of exercise is long-lasting (at least 24 h), but likely diminishes with increasing time post-exercise." While the anabolic effect of exercise lasts for 24 hours or more, the maximum anabolic effect occurs during the first 2-4 hours after exercise. This is why a post-workout supplement is generally recommended immediately following a workout. Because there is a limit to how much protein can be consumed at one time, additional protein should be consumed at regular intervals over the next 24 hours (recommendation #6).

#8: "While it is possible for physically active individuals to obtain their daily protein requirements through the consumption of whole foods, supplementation is a practical way of ensuring intake of adequate protein quality and quantity, while minimizing caloric intake."

#9: "Rapidly digested proteins that contain high proportions of essential amino acids and adequate leucine are most effective in stimulating muscle protein synthesis." This recommendation is most appropriate for protein(s) ingested during the acute 2-4-hour anabolic phase immediately after exercise. During the remaining 24 hours of the anabolic phase, it is more important to maintain a constant amino acid concentration in the bloodstream. For this reason,

I generally recommend more slowly digested proteins, such as meat or soy, between 4 and 24 hours after exercise.

#10: "Different types and quality of protein can affect amino acid bioavailability following protein supplementation." Simply put, there are a lot of "junk" protein supplements out there. Look for a manufacturer with a reputation for integrity and for product quality. Integrity and product quality are issues I will cover in my upcoming book "Slaying the Supplement Myths".

#11: "Athletes should consider focusing on whole food sources of protein that contain all the essential amino acids." Simply put, you should avoid supplements that contain only a few selected amino acids. Instead, choose supplements that provide whole protein from natural sources. Leucine, for example, is very beneficial when added to a whole protein supplement containing all the essential amino acids, but leucine by itself would be of little value.

#12: "Endurance athletes should focus on achieving adequate carbohydrate intake to promote optimal performance; the addition of protein may help offset muscle damage and promote recovery." In short, endurance athletes benefit from a combination of carbohydrates and protein, but carbohydrates are of primary importance.

#13: "Pre-sleep casein intake (30-40 g) provides increases in overnight muscle protein synthesis and metabolic rate without decreasing the overnight fat breakdown." The definitive studies on this have been fairly recent. This recommendation is most appropriate for elite athletes who are primarily interested in increasing muscle mass. For the rest of us, calorie considerations would outweigh the small increment in muscle mass we could gain overnight.

Summary

The oft repeated statement that most Americans are getting too much protein and that excess protein is harmful is a myth. It would be correct to say that most Americans are getting too much of the wrong kinds of protein (fatty animal proteins) and those proteins are harmful to our health. We should be eating more plant proteins. It would also be correct to say that the average middle-aged couch potatoes among us are probably getting more protein than we need. However, many other groups may not be getting enough protein in their diet. The increased protein needs of teenage girls, pregnant women and lactating women have been long recognized, and are incorporated into existing RDAs, but teenage girls and pregnant and lactating women often don't meet those protein RDAs. Moreover, recent research suggests that seniors, dieters, and athletes have increased protein needs in the range of 1.5-2 times the current RDA. Many of those individuals with increased protein needs are not getting enough protein in their diet. This is especially true for seniors and dieters.

Food Myth #7: Red Meat Madness

We love meat in this country. Like most of you, I grew up eating steak and potatoes, burgers and fries, and fried chicken and hush puppies. Summer holidays and special events were always celebrated with "pig pickings." (As you might have guessed, I grew up in the south). Just like many of you, meat was part of my cultural heritage. Because of that, I understand how hard it is to even conceive that meat might be bad for us. Ingrained habits and beliefs are hard to change. I think that goes a long way toward explaining why recommendations to limit red meat consumption have been so controversial.

As I mention earlier, the controversy started in the 50s and 60s when Dr. Ancel Keys showed that saturated fats increased your risk of heart disease. About the same time, the Framingham Heart Study showed that cholesterol was bad for us. Suddenly, those delicious marbled steaks became a "no-no." Then we learned that processed meats were bad for us. That meant that meats like bacon, sausage, hot dogs, bologna, and salami were on the "naughty list." What were we to eat for breakfast and lunch? The final straw came when the experts started recommending that we replace some of the meat in our diet with plant-based proteins like beans and legumes. That was blasphemy. You mean beans and vegetables were actually a meal?

An insurgency was born. Everyone loves opposing those dumb scientists and government health agencies. What do they know? The mantra became: don't worry about saturated fats and cholesterol. Don't give up your meats. Give up carbs instead. If we were just talking about refined carbohydrates and sugar, most nutrition experts would have no concerns with low-carb diets. However, most of the low-carb diets also eliminate plant-based protein sources because they also contain carbohydrates. That leaves these diets heavily dependent on meat as the major source of protein.

If we are talking about fatty cuts of meat, that is a clear problem because, as we discussed previously, saturated fat and cholesterol increase the risk of heart disease. But, what if we only consumed lean cuts of beef and pork? Better yet, what if we ate only grass-fed beef, as recommended in some of the newer low-carb diets? Grass-fed beef is lower in fat, lower in saturated fat, and has a healthier ratio of omega-3 to omega-6 polyunsaturated fats. Is that OK? Possibly, but I still have one big concern – cancer.

The International Agency For Research On Cancer (IARC), the agency created by the WHO to set international standards for cancer risk, has designated red meat as a class 2a ***carcinogen***. That designation means that there is probable cause to believe that it increases cancer risk in humans. The evidence is best for increased risk of colon cancer and breast cancer, although there is some evidence that it may also increase risk of pancreatic and prostate cancer.

The increased cancer risk of red meat does not seem to be solely due to its fat content, so grass-fed beef is just as likely to increase cancer risk as conventionally raised beef. There are multiple proposed mechanisms for this effect:

- When fat and juices from the meat drip onto an open flame, carcinogenic polyaromatic hydrocarbons are formed that stick to the surface of the meat. This can be reduced, but not eliminated, by lower fat meat choices. Some studies suggest they can also be reduced by marinating the meat prior to cooking.
- When red meats are cooked at high temperatures, amino acids in the meat combine with a compound called creatine, which is found in all red meats, to form carcinogenic heterocyclic amines. This can be reduced by cooking the meat at lower temperatures.
- Heme iron, which is found in all red meats, combines with amino acids in the meat to form carcinogenic N-nitroso compounds in our intestines. This mechanism is inherent in all red meats and cannot be eliminated by choosing lower fat cuts or cooking at lower temperatures.
- People who eat high-meat diets have an entirely different population of intestinal bacteria than people who eat no meat. Several recent studies suggest that the intestinal bacteria of meat eaters are more likely to convert the foods we eat into chemicals that increase the risk of cancer and heart disease. I gave one example earlier, namely that creatine is metabolized differently in the intestines of meat-eaters and vegetarians, and the metabolite created in the intestines of meat-eaters may increase the risk of heart disease.

To be clear, red meat is only a probable carcinogen and we aren't sure of the exact mechanism(s) that cause this ***carcinogenicity***. We do not yet have definitive evidence that red meat causes cancer. However, there is good reason to be cautious about how much red meat we consume.

The good news is that the antioxidants, fiber and phytonutrients found in fruits and vegetables can block most of these cancer-causing pathways. Specifically:

- The fiber found in fruits, vegetables and whole grains binds to polyaromatic hydrocarbons and heterocyclic amines and flushes them through the intestines.
- Polyaromatic hydrocarbons require activation by the liver before they become carcinogenic. Indoles and isothiocyanates found in broccoli, cabbage, and other cruciferous vegetables inhibit the enzymes that catalyze this activation.
- Antioxidants found in fruits, vegetables and whole grains reduce the formation of N-nitroso compounds in the intestines.
- A largely plant-based diet appears to favor a population of intestinal bacteria that is less likely to convert compounds in meat into cancer-causing chemicals. [Note: This is a new area of research, so the data supporting this mechanism of cancer prevention are less definitive than for the other three mechanisms.]

This means that small amounts of red meat in a largely plant-based diet may not be as concerning. Specifically, an ounce of red meat in a large green salad or stir fry is much less likely to increase your cancer risk than a 6-ounce steak with fries. Of course, it would be even healthier if you substituted chicken, fish, or legumes for the red meat.

This may also explain why diets such as Mediterranean and DASH that include fruits, vegetables and whole grains with small amounts of meat appear to be healthier than the low-carb diets that emphasize meat and often restrict fruits and whole grains. This will be covered in much more detail in the next chapter.

Food Myth #8: Organic Obsession

Organic and non-GMO are "in," and the marketing departments of all your favorite food and food supplement companies know it. Consequently, you are seeing more and more foods and food supplements labeled "Certified Organic" and "Certified non-GMO." But do those labels guarantee that the products are purer and safer? Maybe not.

Don't misunderstand me. There are plenty of very good reasons to choose foods that are organic and non-GMO. However, like many other aspects of the food and food supplement industries, the myths have outgrown the realities. Once again, food and food supplement companies are only too happy to promise us what we want even if what we've asked for is unscientific, and the product claims are untrue. Let's start with "Certified Organic" and ask which claims are true and which are not.

Are Organic Foods Pure?

When a food is certified organic that means that it is grown without chemical fertilizers, pesticides and herbicides. That is a good reason to choose organic whenever possible, but it is no guarantee of purity. Unfortunately, we live in a very contaminated world. Pesticides and herbicides can be carried by the wind from surrounding farms. More frequently, pesticides and herbicides from neighboring farms contaminate the groundwater and are taken up by the organically grown plants without the farmer's knowledge. Even more alarming, much of the world's groundwater is contaminated with industrial chemicals and heavy metals.

For example, a recent meta-analysis[63] combined the results of 343 of the best-designed previous studies comparing organic and conventionally grown crops. The good news was:

- Pesticide residues were four-fold lower in the organically raised produce than in the conventionally raised produce. This result has been consistently seen in most previously published studies, and is probably the #1 reason that people choose organic produce.
- Polyphenol antioxidant levels were also significantly higher in the organically raised produce. The percent increase ranged from 19% to 69% depending on the polyphenolic compound tested. This increase has not been seen in all previously published studies, but would represent a side benefit if true.
- Increased levels of vitamins and minerals were seen for organically raised foods in some studies, but this was not a consistent finding.

The bad news was:

- Pesticide contamination of organically raised foods was not zero in any of the 343 studies. Consumers are led to believe that organic foods are free of pesticide contamination. They are not. They are simply less contaminated than conventionally raised foods.
- Arsenic and lead contamination was identical in organically and conventionally raised foods. That is because heavy metal contamination comes from groundwater and has nothing to do with how the crops are raised. This study did not look at contamination with industrial

chemicals, but they would also likely contaminate organically and conventionally raised foods equally.

Groundwater contamination is the "elephant in the room" that the organic food industry is not talking about. The problem is that testing of organic foods, when it is done, focuses on pesticides and herbicides. Nobody is testing for groundwater contaminants. That means that most suppliers and manufacturers have no idea how contaminated their organic foods and food products are.

Let me give you two examples from a recent conversation I had with the head of Research and Development of a very reputable food supplement manufacturer.

Example #1: His company was looking for an organic source of tea leaves for a new product they were developing. He was told by his contacts in the industry that the absolute best source of organic tea leaves was a remote farm region in India. When he checked it out, he found that his contacts were correct. The villagers used manure for fertilizer. They used no pesticides or herbicides. Their tea leaves were certified organic.

However, he decided to practice due diligence. He purchased samples of the tea leaves and brought them back to the company's laboratories for analysis. The leaves turned out to be the most contaminated ingredient they had ever tested! After a bit of sleuthing he discovered that there was a major industrial complex 30 miles away, and it had thoroughly contaminated the groundwater. The farmers had done their best. Their tea leaves were certified organic, but they were far from pure!

Example #2: His company was considering expanding their product offerings in the area of protein supplements, so he decided to do a little market research. He went to a local retailer and purchased several protein products and brought them back to the laboratory for analysis. One of the protein supplement labels claimed to be certified organic, certified non-GMO, and certified fair trade. It sounded fantastic.

What's not to like about a product like that? There was only one problem. When he analyzed it in the laboratory, it was heavily contaminated with lead. In fact, it had 4 times the lead levels allowed by California Proposition 65. It was so contaminated that it should have had a warning label for it to be sold in California.

The problem once again was groundwater contamination. The protein product had a high concentration of rice protein. Rice is particularly susceptible to groundwater pollution because it spends most of the growing season partially submerged in water. Because of that, rice and rice proteins are frequently contaminated with lead and arsenic. This is yet another example of a product that was certified organic, but wasn't pure.

The Bottom Line

While organic foods have less pesticides than conventionally grown foods, the level of those contaminants is not zero – even with organic certification. The problem is that our environment is so polluted that no farm is contaminant free. A farmer can use the best organic practices, but if their groundwater is contaminated or pesticides from neighboring farms blow onto their farm, some of those toxic residues end up in their "organic" crops. When you are buying fruits and vegetables, I recommend buying organic whenever possible. With processed foods and food supplements, the story is more complex. Unfortunately, there are too many manufacturers that simply assume that organic means pure and don't run independent quality control tests to check for purity. For that reason, my advice is to ignore "Certified Organic" labels on processed foods and food supplements and inquire instead about the number and type of quality controls the manufacturer uses to assure that the product is actually pure.

Food Myth #9: Non-GMO Nonsense

Should We Demand All Food Ingredients Be Non-GMO?

Don't misunderstand me. I'm no proponent of genetically modified foods. There are potential risks to genetically modified foods because they contain foreign DNA, and there are potential risks to proteins derived from genetically modified foods because of possible food allergies to the foreign protein those foods contain. However, non-GMO proponents start to move beyond what good science supports when they also assert there are health risks to food ingredients (sugars, oils, and the like) purified from genetically modified foods. Those food ingredients contain no DNA and no protein. They contain no genetic information. They are chemically and biologically indistinguishable whether they come from GM or non-GM sources.

So, with respect to the question of whether we should demand that all ingredients be non-GMO, my answer is a clear no. For that reason, I'm no fan of some the proposed GMO labeling laws that do not distinguish between non-GMO foods and non-GMO food ingredients. I am also no fan of the "Certified Non-GMO" label on processed foods and food supplements because it requires manufacturers to certify that all ingredients are non-GMO, even those ingredients for which non-GMO sourcing makes no difference. That adds extra cost to the product and provides no benefit to the consumer.

I do recommend that we buy non-GMO fruits, vegetables and grains. I also recommend we buy processed foods and food supplements that contain non-GMO proteins. I consider it a waste of money to buy non-GMO oils, sugars, and other nutrients that have been purified from foods. For processed foods and food supplements the "Certified Non-GMO" label is overkill. I would like to see non-GMO labeling that pertained only to those ingredients for which non-GMO sourcing was important. That would be scientifically defensible and would be of real value to the consumer.

Are Non-GMO Foods Pure?

The concern here is about the 100 million pounds/year of Roundup that we are spraying on our crops in this country. What proponents of the non-GMO argument fail to realize is that Roundup is used for both GM and non-GMO crops. It is widely used as a "desiccant" for non-GMO crops like wheat, peas and beans. That simply means that Roundup is sprayed on the fields shortly before harvest. That kills the weeds and causes the leaves to drop off the crop, making mechanical harvesting much more efficient.

The implications of this practice are significant. For GM crops Roundup is used for weed control in early to mid-season. Because Roundup degrades relatively quickly, most of it is gone by the time the crops are harvested. However, when Roundup is used as a desiccant for non-GMO crops, it is applied just before harvest – meaning that some non-GMO crops are more likely to be contaminated than the GM crops.

The bottom line is that non-GMO certification is no guarantee of purity. Once again, stringent quality controls by your processed food or food supplement company are always your best guarantee of purity.

This was a very simplistic discussion of the myths surrounding GM versus non-GMO foods and food products. For a more detailed analysis of the controversies around GM foods, see my video "The Truth About Genetically Modified Foods" on the video resource page of https://healthtipsfromtheprofessor.com.

Food Myth #10: Label Lunacy

I get a lot of questions about food ingredient labels. That's because in today's internet world everyone is an "expert" wanting to be heard. Couple that with the fact that old news is boring, and we have a problem. All these "experts" have to keep coming up with new information that is novel and scary. It doesn't need to be true – just novel and scary.

The warnings about which food ingredients to avoid are a perfect example. A few years ago, it was simple to know which ingredients to avoid. If you avoided foods with sugar, refined flour, trans fats and all that artificial stuff, you were OK. However, in recent years the list of ingredients to avoid keeps getting longer and longer.

It has reached the point where it is getting hard to find a food product or food supplement that doesn't have any of the ingredients on the "naughty list." You may even be wondering if there is anything besides organic fresh fruits and vegetables that you can actually eat. How did we get to this point?

The answer is obvious. All the internet "experts" needed something new to warn us about so they took molehills and turned them into mountains. They took food ingredients that might cause a few problems for a limited number of people and characterized them as ingredients that were dangerous for everyone. Their posts were picked up and repeated by other "experts" and soon everyone thought they had to be true. The warnings about food ingredients became "urban nutrition myths."

It is time for a myth buster to come along and help you sort through all the ingredient warnings so that you know which ones are true and which are myths. Let me be your guide.

I began my "research" by Googling "Food Ingredients to Avoid" to see what was on the internet. After a bit of "research" I came up with 25 of the most frequently mentioned "dangerous" food ingredients and have divided them into 3 categories. I call them "The Good, The Bad and the Ugly."

Food Ingredients: The Good

Let me start by identifying the "good ones" – those food ingredients that are on many of the internet "naughty lists," but are actually OK for most people most of the time. I would be the first to admit that using the word "good" as a descriptor for food ingredients is a bit of a misnomer. The word "good" should really be reserved for organic fresh fruits and vegetables along with other whole, unprocessed foods. Of course, the problem is that most of us don't eat enough of those foods, so we need to know which ingredients in the processed foods and food supplements we eat are OK.

The list of food ingredients that are perfectly OK for most of us would be a long one, so let me just mention a few that have inadvertently slipped onto the online "naughty lists" that you may have seen.

GMO: As I said before, I am no fan of GMO foods, but ingredients derived from GMO foods are a very different story. I have covered this topic in detail in the previous section, so let me just summarize the key points here.

- GMO foods and proteins derived from GMO foods can be a problem because of food sensitivities to the modified proteins. That risk is real, but it's difficult to quantify.
- All other food ingredients derived from genetically modified foods contain no genetic information or proteins. They are chemically and biologically indistinguishable from the same ingredients derived from non-GMO foods. Consequently, there are no health risks associated with these food ingredients.
- I am aware of the recent internet chatter about the WHO declaring that Roundup can cause cancer. However, as I pointed out earlier, some non-GMO foods are more

likely to be contaminated with Roundup residues than are GMO foods.

- That just leaves the environmental issue. Roundup does break down relatively quickly in the environment, but I do have concerns about spraying tons of the stuff on our crops every year. However, I must acknowledge that many of my scientific colleagues do not share this concern, and they are not all in bed with Monsanto.

Soy: I cover this topic in detail in my upcoming book, "Slaying the Supplement Myths," so I will just summarize briefly here.

- The myths that soy consumption causes breast cancer or any other cancer, lowers testosterone levels in men, and interferes with thyroid metabolism have been disproven by multiple clinical studies.
- The idea that soy must be fermented to be healthy is a myth. Most soy products are processed in such a manner that toxins in the soy bean are removed.
- For ingredients made from soy such as soy lecithin, there are no health risks associated with sourcing them from GMO soy (see my discussion about GMO). If you are consuming a soy protein product, however, I do recommend that you choose non-GMO soy.

Carrageenan: Carrageenan comes from seaweed and red algae. It has been used in foods for thousands of years because of its gelling properties. In the supplement world, it is used to improve consistency and the disintegration of tablets. There is a lot to like about carrageenan. It is natural, organic and non-GMO. Why then has it become an internet villain in the food ingredient world? The problem is that most of the internet "experts" who are vilifying carrageenan are not distinguishing between carrageenan and its breakdown product poligeenan. Here are the facts:

- In some animal studies poligeenan at very high doses has been shown to cause diarrhea, hemorrhaging and ulcerations of the colon and even colon cancer. Not all animal studies agree, but this does raise the possibility that high doses of poligeenan might cause the same effects in humans.
- Food grade carrageenan contains <5% poligeenan and does not raise the same concerns.
- Food grade carrageenan does not cause gastrointestinal problems in most animal studies. Nor has it been shown to cause cancer in any animal study.
- The FDA, USDA and WHO have reviewed all available studies and have concluded that food grade carrageenan is safe.
- The International Agency for Research on Cancer (IARC) has concluded that carrageenan does not cause cancer.

Caramel Color: I won't go into detail here, but the argument is similar to that for carrageenan. It is a minor impurity of caramel coloring that is the concern. However, caramel coloring itself should not be a concern for products made by any reputable manufacturer that employs rigorous quality control tests on their ingredients.

Canola Oil: Canola oil is an excellent source of monounsaturated fats and polyunsaturated fats, especially the beneficial omega-3 polyunsaturated fats. In supplements, it is primarily used as a source of healthy fats and to improve taste, aroma or texture. There are some legitimate concerns with canola oil, but they have been considerably overhyped. This is a perfect example of a molehill being turned into a mountain. Let's look at the myths that are simply untrue and the facts that have been overhyped.

Myth #1: Canola oil contains the same toxins as the original rapeseed oil. Fact: The toxins found in rapeseed oil have been removed through conventional plant breeding. Canola oil is toxin free.

Myth #2: Canola oil is toxic in animal studies. Fact: When you look at those studies carefully they were either done with rapeseed oil or were done under conditions where almost any vegetable oil would have been problematic.

Fact #1: Canola oil is highly processed. That's true, but so are most other vegetable oils. If you want a less processed oil, choose virgin olive oil.

Fact #2: Most canola oil comes from GMO plants. That is true, but canola oil is a highly purified food ingredient. As described previously, that means there are no health concerns from eating GMO canola oil, only a possible environmental concern.

Maltodextrin: Maltodextrin is a natural food ingredient made from enzymatically digesting starch. It is used as a stabilizer and thickener in foods. It is also combined with glucose and fructose in sports drinks to provide sustained energy.

Myth #1: The internet is filled with claims that maltodextrin causes gastrointestinal problems or that it is unsafe. There is very little evidence to back that up, and we need to consider those claims in light of the fact that we produce lots of maltodextrin in our intestines every day as we digest the starches in our diet.

Myth #2: "Maltodextrin is just another sugar. It is just another way for food manufacturers to hide the total amount of sugar in their products." Maltodextrin is actually less sweet than most sugars. As described above, it is primarily added to foods for reasons other than to impart sweetness.

Fact: Most of the maltodextrin in the US does come from GMO corn. Once again, it is a highly purified food ingredient. As with canola oil, that means there are no health concerns, only possible environmental concerns.

Carmine (also known as cochineal): I find this one truly amusing. Websites breathlessly proclaim: "Did you know that the red dye used in your favorite food comes from ground-up insects?" Of course, the statement is factually correct. Carmine is a red food dye extracted and purified from a tropical beetle. However, the implication the statement suggests is completely misleading. This is a highly purified ingredient. It contains no insect parts. In fact, you are far more likely to find insect parts in your breakfast cereal or piece of toast. The FDA allows up to 350 insect fragments, 5 rodent hairs, and 2 rodent poop pellets in every cup of flour. Enjoy your breakfast cereal and toast!

Carmine dye is natural, organic, and non-GMO. It is much safer than the Red #2 or Red #40 it replaces. What's not to like? Are the alarmists worried that the beetles will become an endangered species or are they concerned about the suffering of the beetles who give up their lives to produce carmine dye?

Food Ingredients: The Bad

The term "bad" for the food ingredients in this list is also a bit of a misnomer. In some cases, these are food ingredients that a few people should avoid, but which are perfectly OK for many people. In other cases, the type of food the ingredients are added to determines whether the ingredient is OK or should be avoided. However, these are nuances that seem to escape the average internet blogger.

Sodium Nitrate and Nitrite: This is a perfect example of a food ingredient that can be "bad" in certain foods and "good" in others. Briefly:

- When sodium nitrate and/or sodium nitrite are added to processed meats, they can combine with the amino acids from the meat in the intestines to form cancer-causing nitrosamines. As you might suspect, this is not a good thing.
- On the other hand, when sodium nitrate or sodium nitrite are found in fruits and vegetables or combined with natural antioxidants such as vitamin C in food supplements, they are converted to nitric oxide, which has many beneficial effects in the body.

Sugar and High Fructose Corn Syrup: As I said earlier, there are no sugar villains and there are no sugar heroes. The problems associated with sugars of all types in the American diet are related to the amount of sugar in our diet (too much) and the kinds of foods they are found in. In summary:

- When sugars are consumed as a part of foods that are rich in fiber and/or protein they have much less of an effect on blood sugar levels (a lower glycemic index) than when they are consumed in sodas, juices and highly processed foods. That's important because the bad health consequences of sugars are primarily caused by foods that lead to high blood sugar levels.
- Consequently, we should be focusing on the glycemic index (the effect on blood sugar levels) of the foods we eat rather than obsessing about the amount or kinds of sugar on the label.

MSG: MSG, or monosodium glutamate, is a particularly interesting case. MSG is the sodium salt of the amino acid glutamate. Glutamate is found in every protein in our body and in every protein we eat. However, glutamate is also a neurotransmitter. That poses a problem for some people:

- When MSG is used as a flavor enhancer in foods with a low-protein content, the glutamate is very rapidly taken up by the brain and can overstimulate some neurons.
    - For most people this is no problem, but a small number of people experience what used to be called "Chinese Restaurant Syndrome" due to the large amounts of MSG used in some Chinese foods.
    - The common symptoms associated with "Chinese Restaurant Syndrome" are headache, sweating, skin flushing, nausea and fatigue. Allergic reactions to MSG can even be life threatening in some individuals.

Because of that, MSG is no longer widely used as a flavor enhancer, and most restaurants either no longer use it or provide warning labels so sensitive individuals can avoid foods containing MSG. However, now the internet bloggers are warning you to avoid foods containing hydrolyzed or enzymatically digested vegetable protein and sodium caseinate because they contain MSG. That is utter nonsense.

- Glutamate is one of the 20 amino acids found in every protein we eat. As that protein is digested in our intestines, monosodium glutamate (MSG) is released. Hydrolyzed vegetable protein and sodium caseinate are simply pre-digested proteins. They contain no more MSG than we would have produced if we digested them ourselves.
- Monosodium glutamate (MSG) formed during the digestion of a complete protein is no more dangerous than any of the other amino acids released during digestion of that protein. That is because when all the amino acids are in the blood at the same time, they compete with glutamate for uptake into the brain. This

slows the entry of glutamate into the brain and prevents overstimulation of neurons.

The bottom line is that MSG as a flavor enhancer is harmless for most people, but problematic for some. MSG as a component of hydrolyzed vegetable protein or sodium caseinate is harmless for everyone because it is in balance with the other naturally occurring amino acids.

Salt (Sodium): I could, and probably should, write a whole article on sodium intake. Suffice it to say that 1) most of us consume too much sodium, 2) most of that sodium is hidden in the foods we eat rather than added at the table, and 3) some people are more sensitive to the bad effects of sodium than others.

Refined Grains: Again, this could be a whole article. Suffice it to say that 1) whole grains are better than refined grains and 2) most of us would benefit from eating fewer refined grains and more fruits and vegetables in their place.

Food Ingredients: The Ugly

Finally, there are some food ingredients that most experts (except for those in the food industry) agree should be avoided. I call them the dirty dozen. They are:

1) Trans fats (also known as partially hydrogenated vegetable oils)
2) Aspartame
3) Acesulfame K
4) Sucralose
5) Artificial colors
6) Artificial flavors

7) BHA and BHT
8) Propyl gallate
9) Sodium and potassium benzoate
10) Potassium bromate
11) Potassium sorbate
12) Polysorbate 80

Summary – Food Myths Busted

Let's close this section with a summary of the truth about the food myths you have been hearing:

1) Sorry to disappoint you, but eating chocolate is not going to help you lose weight. I included this in the top 10 only because it was an excellent example of how studies that measure associations between diet and health outcomes can mislead.
2) Forget scouring labels for sugars you must avoid. We do need to decrease the total amount of sugar in our diet, but there are no sugar heroes and there are no sugar villains. It's foods that are important, not the sugar they contain. Avoid sugar-sweetened beverages, sugary junk foods, and sugar-laden desserts and pastries. Instead choose foods where the sugar content is balanced with fiber and protein so that the sugar enters our bloodstream slowly (has a low glycemic index).
3) Leave diet sodas and sugar-free diet foods on the shelf. They are not the solution to obesity that the food industry would have you believe. There is no good evidence that diet sodas and diet foods help you lose weight and some evidence they may actually cause you to gain weight. There is also increasing evidence they may

be harmful to your health. Choose water and herbal teas instead of sodas. If you crave carbonation, drink carbonated water. If you crave taste, infuse your water with your favorite fruit. If it is caffeine you crave, choose regular tea or coffee without added sweetener or cream. The transition may be difficult, but a couple of months from now your taste buds and your body will thank you for making healthier choices.

4) The evidence has become overwhelming that saturated fats increase your risk of dying from heart disease. I endorse the American Heart Association recommendation to consume moderate amounts of fat and replace at least half of the saturated fat in your diet with monounsaturated fat and polyunsaturated fat. The American Heart Association's data show that if you do that in the context of a heart-healthy diet of fresh fruits, vegetables and whole grains such as the Mediterranean diet, you can cut your risk of heart disease in half.

5) Ignore the coconut oil craze. There is currently no good evidence that it is bad for you, but there is also no good evidence that it is good for you. My advice is: If you have a favorite recipe for which coconut oil provides the perfect flavor, go ahead and use it. Just don't go out of your way to use it in all your cooking. We may find out a few years down the road that it is as bad for us as some health experts claim.

6) Ignore claims that we are eating too much protein and it is going to do dreadful things to us. The claim that we are eating too much protein primarily applies to middle-aged couch potatoes. Many other groups, such as teenage girls, pregnant and lactating women, seniors, dieters, and athletes and fitness enthusiasts, may not be getting enough protein from our diet. What is true is that we are eating too much of the wrong kind of

protein. We should be eating less fatty meats, and more plant-based proteins such as beans and other legumes.

7) We love our red meat in this country, but we should ignore the siren call of those "gurus" who tell us we can eat as much as we like. Fatty meats dramatically increase our risk of heart disease. Even lean meats and grass-fed beef may pose problems. Red meat is considered a class 2a carcinogen, which means it is a probable cause of cancer. Fortunately, a diet rich in fruits, vegetables, and whole grains can neutralize some of the carcinogenic properties of meat. Consequently, small amounts of meat in a primarily plant-based diet may be OK.

8) We should choose organic fruits and vegetables whenever possible. However, we live in a polluted world. Consequently, we need to understand that organic does not mean pure. Organic fruits and vegetables contain less pesticides and herbicides than conventionally raised crops, but their level is not zero. Even worse, organic certification does not measure groundwater contamination. Some organic crops are heavily contaminated with heavy metals and industrial chemicals from groundwater. For prepared foods and food supplements, the quality control standards of the manufacturer are more important than "Certified Organic" on the label.

9) Non-GMO certification is important for whole foods and proteins derived from whole foods. However, it is meaningless when applied to nutrients (oils, sugars, etc.) that have been purified from food sources because they contain no protein and no genetic information. They are chemically and biologically identical whether obtained from GMO or non-GMO crops. Non-GMO is also no guarantee of purity. Some non-GMO crops are sprayed with Roundup just prior to harvesting to improve the efficiency of mechanical harvesting. They

are more likely to be contaminated than GMO crops because when Roundup is used for weed control on GMO crops, spraying must stop 6 weeks prior to harvest.

10) The internet "gurus" are constantly warning you to read your labels carefully because they have discovered another ingredient that is bad for you. You can ignore most of those warnings. They are bogus. I reviewed the top 25 and told you which warnings were true and which you can ignore.

4

Dueling Diets

Diets are a lot like politics in today's world. Everyone is absolutely convinced their diet is the best and absolutely convinced the other diets are terrible. Remember the nursery rhyme: "Jack Sprat could eat no fat. His wife could eat no lean…"? Today's diets remind me of that. They run the gamut from no fat to no carbohydrates. Surely, both extremes can't be healthy. Or can they? Some diets eliminate whole food groups. That can't be a good thing. Or, can it?

How To Evaluate Diets

In this chapter, I will give you the pros and cons of these dueling diets. Before I do that, however, let me give you some principles to put things into perspective. I have mentioned some of these things before, but they bear repeating before we take a deep dive into an analysis of dueling diets.

We are omnivores. We can adapt to a wide variety of diets and do reasonably well. That means most people will do well on any of these diets short-term.

Anything is better than the standard American diet (SAD). It is high in sugar and refined carbohydrates. It is also high in saturated and trans fats. That is why proponents of every diet can claim that you will feel better and be healthier when you switch to their diet.

Processed and convenience foods are a big part of the problem. Most diets recommend "clean eating" (elimination of processed and convenience foods). Any diet that eliminates processed and convenience foods is likely to help you lose weight and get healthier. **Caution**: As soon as a diet becomes popular, food manufacturers rush in to provide pre-packaged, convenience foods to support that diet. Avoid the temptation to use those foods. Big Food Inc does not have your best interests in mind. They are not your friends.

Most diets lead to a fairly rapid initial weight loss. There are several reasons for this:

- Most diets eliminate sodas, fast foods and junk foods. That alone leads to significant weight loss.
- There is the psychological aspect. Most people focus much more carefully on what they eat during the early stages of a new diet.
- Low-carb diets cause water loss. The water weight comes back as soon as you add carbs back to the diet.
- Many diets restrict food choices. Often, they eliminate whole food groups. When you eliminate familiar foods from someone's diet, they instinctively eat less without even thinking about it.

This rapid initial weight loss is part of the allure of almost every diet program. However, over time most people start adding back some of their favorite foods or find new foods they like, and the weight comes back.

Weight loss leads to improved blood parameters irrespective of diet composition. That is why every diet, no matter how bizarre, can claim it lowers your blood pressure, improves your blood sugar, lowers your cholesterol, and lowers your triglycerides.

Long-term weight loss is virtually identical on every diet. Numerous clinical studies have compared long-term weight loss on low-fat diets, low-carbohydrate diets, and virtually everything in between. Initial weight loss is more rapid on the low-carbohydrate diets. However, at the end of one or two years there is not a dime's worth of difference in weight loss between any of the diets. The exception is a vegetarian diet. Vegetarians typically weigh less than their meat-eating counterparts, probably because the foods in the vegetarian diet have lower caloric density (fewer calories per serving).

Saturated and trans fats are not your friends. They increase your risk of heart disease. They also increase inflammation, which can have many serious long-term health consequences. In addition, the foods that are rich in saturated fats are often acid-forming foods, which can upset your acid-base balance.

Healthy carbs and healthy fats are more important than low-carb or low-fat diets. Ignore the claims and counter claims about low-fat and low-carb diets. Focus instead on diets that provide moderate amounts of whole grains instead of refined grains and sugar. Also focus on diets that provide moderate amounts of monounsaturated and polyunsaturated fats, especially the omega-3 polyunsaturated fats, instead of saturated and trans fats.

Focus on well-balanced meals rather than individual foods. For example, moderate amounts of healthy carbohydrates will have relatively little effect on blood sugar and triglyceride levels as part of a plant-based meal that provides plenty of fiber and protein. However, those same carbohydrate-rich foods by themselves may cause a spike in both blood sugar and triglycerides.

Plant-based diets rule. A vegetarian diet is the only diet that has been shown to reverse atherosclerosis in some people. A vegetarian diet and the Mediterranean and DASH diets, which are largely plant-based, have been shown to be healthy long term. On the other hand, we simply don't know whether the meat-based, low-carbohydrate diets are healthy long term. The little evidence we do have suggests they are less healthy than plant-based diets.

We have 5 food groups for a reason. Each food group provides valuable nutrients (vitamins and minerals) and phytonutrients. You may be able to replace the missing nutrients with supplementation, but you are unlikely to replace the phytonutrients with supplements – even those supplements that claim to be made from whole foods. You should be concerned about the long-term health consequences of any diet that eliminates whole food groups.

Low-fat diets aren't necessarily healthy. Whole food, low-fat diets like the vegan diet are extremely healthy. However, as soon as health experts started recommending low-fat diets, Big Food Inc stepped in to offer convenient low-fat options. They simply replaced the fat with refined carbohydrates, sugar, and a witch's brew of chemicals. (Remember the part about Big Food Inc not being your friend?) As a result, the low-fat diet consumed by most Americans is anything but healthy.

The supposed advantages of low-carbohydrate diets are misleading. Low-carbohydrate diets look very good when you compare them to the Big Food Inc version of the low-fat diet. However, when you compare them to something like the Mediterranean diet, the DASH diet, or a vegetarian diet the advantages disappear.

Avoid sugar-sweetened and diet beverages. This should go without saying. Choose water or herbal teas instead. Add carbonation and/or a little lemon or lime juice for flavoring if necessary. Fortunately, most of the major diets exclude sugar-sweetened and diet beverages.

With these principles in mind, let's take a deep dive into the diet controversy. We will look at diets ranging from the Jack Sprat variety (almost no fat) to his wife (almost all fat). That's a humorous way of saying I will start with vegetarian diets and end with the keto diet.

Do Vegetarians Live Longer?

"Vegetarians don't live longer, it just seems that way." Many of you have probably heard that joke, but is it true? Are vegetarians healthier? Do they live longer? Is meat going to kill you? Let's take a deep dive into the pros and cons of vegetarianism.

Vegetarianism encompasses a wide range of diets. At one extreme is the vegan diet. Vegans eat only plant-derived foods. They don't eat fish, meat, milk, eggs, or honey. It also goes without saying they eat only whole foods (whole grains, plant proteins, fruits and vegetables) and avoid things like sodas, sugary foods, junk foods, and convenience foods. The most extreme form of veganism, popularized by such recent movies as "Eating You Alive" and "What the Health," also eliminates all oils. This keeps fat at <10% of total calories.

To avoid confusion, I will refer to this as a "very low-fat vegan diet." I will use the term "vegan diet" to refer to the more common veganism that includes vegetable oils in the diet. The regular vegan diet is still 100% plant-based. It is also still relatively low in fat, generally in the 20-30% range. Since the fat comes from plants, it is predominantly the healthy monounsaturated and polyunsaturated fats.

Lacto-ovo vegetarians add low-fat dairy foods and eggs to a plant-based diet. The Ornish diet is a modified lacto-ovo vegetarian diet that eliminates all oils and keeps fat at $<10\%$ of calories. Pesco-vegetarians add fish to a plant-based diet, and semi-vegetarians add limited amounts of meat to a plant-based diet.

Do Vegetarian Diets Reverse Atherosclerosis?

Let me start with studies on the very low-fat vegan and Ornish diets. In addition to the diets themselves, both programs emphasize regular exercise and stress reduction practices. Adherents to both plans generally achieve a serum total cholesterol of 150 or less. The Ornish diet and lifestyle program was designed to reduce the risk of cardiovascular disease, and it has been very well studied from that perspective.

In studies of patients with severe ***atherosclerosis*** (clogged arteries) for periods of up to 5 years, the Ornish program resulted in a significant reduction in the degree of atherosclerosis[64-67], inflammation[65], cardiac events[65] (heart attack, stroke, etc.), and cardiac deaths[65-67]. Studies with the very low-fat vegan diet are more limited, but suggest that it also reduces atherosclerosis[68] and cardiac deaths[68,69]. Before moving on to other forms of vegetarianism, let me make the point that those are the only diets that have been shown to reverse atherosclerosis. That is a big deal.

The Seventh-day Adventist Studies

Perhaps the largest group of studies on the health effects of vegetarians has been conducted on the Seventh-day Adventist population located in Southern California. Seventh-day Adventists believe that "God calls us to care for our bodies, treating them with the respect a divine creation deserves." The Adventist church advocates a vegan diet consisting of legumes, whole grains, nuts, fruits, and vegetables. However, it allows personal choice, so a significant number of Adventists choose lacto-ovo vegetarian, pesco-vegetarian, or semi-vegetarian diets.

That diversity has allowed studies of the Adventist population to not only compare a vegetarian diet to the standard American diet of the non-Adventist population living in the same area, but also to compare the various forms of vegetarian diets. Here are a few selected insights gained from these studies (unless otherwise stated, all comparisons are to the non-Adventist population eating the standard American diet):

- Vegetarian diets decrease heart attack risk by 40% in men and 54% in women[70].
- Vegetarian diets decrease cardiovascular deaths by 41% in men and 51% in women[70].
- Diabetes is decreased 62% by a vegan diet, 38% by a lacto-ovo vegetarian diet, and 51% by a semi-vegetarian diet[71].
- Consistent with their effects on diabetes, weight loss was 60% less on a lacto-ovo vegetarian diet than on a vegan diet[72]. Both diets caused significant weight loss compared to the standard American diet.
- Colorectal cancer is decreased 16% on a vegan diet, 18% on a lacto-ovo vegetarian diet, 43% on a pesco-vegetarian diet, and 8% on a semi-vegetarian diet[73]. The greater effectiveness of the pesco-vegetarian diet at reducing colorectal cancer risk is probably due to the addition of long chain omega-3 fatty acids to what is already a very healthy diet.

Recent reviews[74-76] of all the pertinent literature on the Seventh-day Adventist population conclude that vegetarians weigh less, have less inflammation, have lower cholesterol levels and have lower risk of diabetes, heart disease, and hypertension than non-vegetarians. Comparing the various forms of vegetarianism, vegan diets appear to offer somewhat greater protection against obesity, hypertension, diabetes, and cardiovascular mortality than lacto-ovo and semi-vegetarian diets[76]. The health benefits of vegetarian diets also seem to be somewhat greater for men than for women. One might speculate that might be because the average American male has a worse diet than the average American female. So, when men adopt a vegetarian diet it may represent a greater improvement.

The reviews also looked at the nutritional adequacy of vegetarian diets. Vegetarian diets in general are very rich in antioxidants, most B vitamins, and polyphenols. Nutrients of concern for vegan diets are vitamin B12, vitamin D, calcium, iron, zinc, and long chain omega-3 fatty acids[74]. Of those, vitamin B12 and long chain omega-3 fatty acids are the ones most likely to require supplementation. Adequate levels of the other nutrients can be achieved by a well-designed vegan diet.

I would add protein to the list. Don't misunderstand me. It is possible to get adequate protein on a vegetarian diet that includes beans and other legumes as a protein source. However, vegan advocates have been telling people they get all the protein they need from broccoli and other vegetables. That is incredibly bad advice, especially for seniors who are likely to suffer from sarcopenia (age-related loss of muscle mass). Broccoli only provides 3 grams of protein per serving. You would need 15 servings to meet the protein RDA for women and almost 19 servings for men. And, as discussed earlier, seniors probably need more than the RDA of protein to prevent sarcopenia (age-related loss of muscle mass)[49]. Unfortunately, I often run across seniors who think they are getting all the protein they need from green salads and steamed vegetables. The bad advice from vegan advocates may be condemning them to unnecessary frailty in their old age.

What about the health claims of the low-carbohydrate diets? Most of those "health benefits" are inferred from changes in blood parameters that occur over the first few weeks or months someone adopts those diets. There are no long-term data showing that low-carbohydrate diets reduce the prevalence of diabetes, heart disease or cancer. Moreover, the few studies that compare low-carbohydrate and vegetarian diets suggest the vegetarian diet is superior. For example, a recent study[77] compared the Atkins diet (the granddaddy of the low-carb diets) with the Ornish diet. People on the low-fat Ornish diet had significantly lower LDL cholesterol, apoB, and C-reactive protein (a marker of inflammation), and had better arterial function than people on the high-fat Atkins diet. I will discuss other studies comparing vegetarian diets with traditional low-carb diets later in this chapter.

Do Vegetarians Live Longer?

What about the original question? Do vegetarians live longer? The answer isn't clear. The Adventist Health Studies have reported that Adventist men live 6-7 years longer and Adventist women live ~4 years longer than their non-Adventist neighbors[78-79]. However, the Adventist population may have other characteristics that contribute to their longevity. I will cover that in the section on "Blue Zones."

In contrast, a recent Australian study[80] concluded that all-cause mortality was virtually identical for vegetarians and non-vegetarians. However, the authors of that study speculated that vegetarians in Australia have become less healthy because they are now consuming more high-sugar processed "vegetarian" foods. Remember what I said about Big Food Inc not being your friend.

There are some additional pros and cons of vegetarianism that don't require clinical studies to validate.

- The most obvious pro is that vegetarianism is good for the environment. Growing fruits and vegetables requires less water, creates less pollution, and creates less greenhouse warming than raising animals. The oft-quoted statistic that raising cattle creates more greenhouse gases than burning fossil fuels is probably not correct, but it is a significant contributor to greenhouse gas production.
- The most obvious con is that a pure vegan diet is difficult to follow, especially if you are also eliminating oils from your diet. You may have trouble finding food you can eat at your favorite restaurant or when visiting friends. Some people also have digestive issues due to the high fiber content of a vegan diet.

What Does This Mean for You?

There are a few simple take-home messages from the research on the various forms of a vegetarian diet:

- The Ornish diet and the very low-fat vegan diet are the only diets shown to reverse atherosclerosis. If you have serious heart disease and would like to minimize your reliance on drugs and surgery, you should consider them. You will, of course, want to let your doctor know what you are doing.
- Vegetarians are leaner and significantly healthier than non-vegetarians.
- Vegans are slightly healthier than lacto-ovo and semi-vegetarians, but even vegetarians who include some dairy, eggs and meat in a primarily plant-based diet are much healthier than most Americans.
- Vegetarians may not live longer, but they do live healthier longer.

There are also several subtle, but equally important, implications from these studies:

1) **You can forget the claims you must be a vegan purist to obtain any health benefits from vegetarianism.** If you watch movies like "Eating You Alive" or "What the Health," you are led to believe you will suffer terrible health consequences if you add any dairy, eggs, or meat to a vegan diet. In fact, the evidence for reversing atherosclerosis is stronger for the Ornish diet, which is a lacto-ovo vegetarian diet, than it is for a pure vegan diet. For several other health outcomes, the vegan diet is slightly more effective, but both lacto-ovo vegetarian and semi-vegetarian diets are much healthier than the standard American diet.

2) **Vegetarian diets are whole food diets.** If you start adding in processed and convenience foods, even if they are labeled "vegan," you are likely to lose all the health benefits of a vegetarian diet.

3) **You can forget claims that you get all the protein you need from vegetables like broccoli.** That is incredibly bad advice which is likely to condemn seniors to unnecessary frailty in old age.

4) **You can forget the claims that you must avoid carbs at all costs.** The proponents of the low-carb diets will tell you that recommendations to limit fat are based on a lie. They tell you that fat is good for you and carbs will cause you to gain weight, increase inflammation, and increase your risk of diabetes, heart disease, and cancer. You are told to avoid grains and any other foods containing carbohydrates, including some fruits and vegetables. The "danger" of carbohydrates is only true for the refined grains, sugary sodas and junk foods in the standard American diet. Vegetarian diets emphasize

whole grains, fruits and vegetables. They are high in carbohydrates and low in fat, and they reduce weight, inflammation, diabetes, heart disease, and some cancers.

5) **You can forget most claims of weight loss**. Most low-carb diets tout rapid initial weight loss. Unfortunately, most of that weight comes back a year or two later. Only vegetarian diets are associated with lower weight over a period of many years.

In summary, a pure vegan diet is probably the healthiest form of vegetarianism, but it is difficult to follow. Vegetarian diets that are primarily plant-based, but contain small amounts of dairy, eggs, or meat are also very healthy, and may be easier for the average American to follow. That leads us into two other very popular, primarily plant-based diets, the Mediterranean diet and the DASH diet, which I will discuss next.

The Mediterranean Diet

If the Mediterranean diet were one of those fad diets you see on the web, the marketing hype might go something like this:

- What if you could reduce your risk of heart disease by almost 50%, and:
- It didn't cost you an extra penny?
- You didn't need to lose weight (although you would probably get even better results if you did)?
- You didn't need to buy a gym membership and start a workout program (although you would probably get even better results if you did)?
- There were absolutely no side effects?

- There were considerable side benefits like reduced risk of type 2 diabetes, high blood pressure, inflammation, and cognitive decline as you aged?

Would you be interested? I'm willing to bet if this were a TV ad, you would be on the edge of your seat. If it were a new "magic" supplement, you might be reaching for your credit card before the ad was over. If it was the latest "miracle" workout machine, you might order it right away.

However, I am not talking about a magic pill or a miracle workout machine. I'm talking about the Mediterranean diet. Interest in the Mediterranean diet began with the observation that people living in the Mediterranean region had significantly lower incidence of common degenerative diseases than people living in Northern Europe and the United States. The Mediterranean diet is probably the best researched diet, and it turns out to be incredibly healthy. Long-term studies show that it significantly reduces the risk of heart disease, diabetes, high blood pressure and stroke, and some cancers. Before we look at the evidence supporting these claims, let's start by looking at the diet itself.

What Is The Mediterranean Diet?

The Mediterranean diet is a largely plant-based diet which emphasizes fresh fruits and vegetables, whole grains, beans, nuts, fish, olive oil, and moderate consumption of red wine. It minimizes red meats, processed meat products, poultry, and full-fat dairy products. Like other healthy diets, it is a whole food diet that does not include sodas or processed and convenience foods. In addition, it is neither a low-fat nor a low-carb diet. It contains moderate amounts of healthy fats and moderate amounts of healthy carbs.

Can You Cut Your Heart Disease Risk In Half?

The evidence is perhaps strongest for the beneficial effect of the Mediterranean diet on heart disease. Let's start by looking at the study behind the recent headlines claiming the Mediterranean diet could cut your heart disease risk in half. This study[81] followed 2583 adults from the region around Athens, Greece for a period of 10 years. The study evaluated the effect of adherence to the Mediterranean diet on heart disease incidence (based on heart attacks, stroke, angina, ischemia, cardiac arrhythmias, and deaths due to heart disease).

As an aside, you might think that everyone in Greece consumes a Mediterranean diet. Unfortunately, our unhealthy Western diet and our fast foods are making inroads in the birthplace of the Mediterranean diet. Because of that, scientists who study the Mediterranean diet have come up with something called the MedDietScore to measure adherence to the diet. The MedDietScore gives positive points based on how often fresh fruits and vegetables, whole grains, beans, nuts, fish and olive oil are consumed. It gives negative points based on how often meats, meat products, poultry, and full-fat dairy products are consumed. For alcohol, modest consumption is considered a positive, with either no or excess alcohol consumption rating a score of 0. The composite score ranges from 0 to 55, with higher values indicating greater adherence to the Mediterranean diet.

Based on adherence to the MedDietScore, the study results were impressive:

- Each 10% increase in adherence to the Mediterranean diet was associated with a 15% decreased risk of developing heart disease during the 10-year study period.
- When they compared participants in the upper third for adherence to the Mediterranean diet to those in the lower third, their risk of developing heart disease was decreased by 47%. That's huge.

However, the results were even more impressive when they looked at the effects of the Mediterranean diet in combination with known risk factors for heart disease.

- For individuals with low adherence to the Mediterranean diet, risk factors such as obesity, high cholesterol, high triglycerides, high blood pressure, diabetes, and inflammation independently increased the risk of developing heart disease. These results are identical to almost every other published study looking at those risk factors.
- However, for individuals with high adherence to the Mediterranean diet, those same risk factors had only small, non-significant effects on the risk of developing heart disease. If this finding is verified by future studies, it would suggest that adherence to a Mediterranean diet has the potential to override risk factors like obesity, diabetes, high blood pressure and elevated cholesterol.

Of course, I would not recommend that you ignore obesity and other cardiovascular risk factors and just focus on following a Mediterranean diet. I'm pretty sure you will get even better results if you get your weight, blood sugar, cholesterol, and blood pressure under control in addition to following a Mediterranean diet.

If this were the only published study showing that adherence to the Mediterranean diet reduces heart disease risk, I would consider it speculative. However, it is only one of several recent studies that have come to a similar conclusion. I will give you one more example, because this study also has some interesting implications.

The study[82] had an interesting design. There were three groups. The first group followed the Mediterranean diet plus they were given free extra-virgin olive oil. The second group followed the Mediterranean diet plus they were given free nuts. The third group followed a low-fat diet.

The low-fat diet was one that is frequently recommended for heart patients. It included low-fat dairy products; bread, potatoes, pasta, and rice; fresh fruits; fresh vegetables; lean fish and seafood. It discouraged commercial baked goods, sweets, and pastries; nuts and fried snacks; red and processed fatty meats; visible fat in meats and soups; fatty fish and seafood canned in oil; spread fats; and vegetable oils (including olive oil). In short, it was a pretty healthy diet.

The study was supposed to go 10 years, but it was cut short at 5 years because the two Mediterranean Groups were doing so much better. In comparison to the low-fat group, stroke and total cardiovascular events were decreased by:

- 30% in the group following the Mediterranean diet plus extra olive oil.
- 28% in the group following the Mediterranean diet plus extra nuts.

In short, the Mediterranean diet was significantly more effective at decreasing heart disease risk than the low-fat diet often recommended for heart disease patients.

The Mediterranean Diet and Other Diseases

At this point in time, the evidence is very strong that following a Mediterranean-type diet will reduce your heart disease risk. However, the Mediterranean diet also appears to reduce the risk of several other diseases.

For example, a recent review[83] of five large prospective clinical trials concluded "The evidence so far accumulated suggests that adopting a Mediterranean diet may help prevent type 2 diabetes. Moreover, a lower carbohydrate, Mediterranean-style diet is good for HbA1c reduction [blood sugar control] in persons with established diabetes."

The Mediterranean diet has also been shown to reduce the risk of several cancers, with the evidence of risk reduction being strongest for breast cancer[84-86] and colon cancer [85,86]. The beneficial effects of the Mediterranean diet on cancer risk appear to be due to increased consumption of fruits and vegetables, fish, whole grains, and olive oil, plus decreased consumption of red meat and refined grains[86]. Recent studies have also suggested that adherence to the Mediterranean diet may reduce the risk of Parkinson's disease[87] and Alzheimer's disease[88]. In addition, for patients who were already diagnosed with Alzheimer's, adherence to the Mediterranean diet increased survival by 3.9 years[89].

In short, long-term clinical studies have shown that the Mediterranean diet is a very healthy diet. While it is different from the usual American diet, it is a diet that most Americans find relatively easy to follow. I should caution, however, that it is not a diet with a lot of pasta. That is a less healthy diet you would find in Northern Italy. This diet is more typical of what you find in other Mediterranean regions – relatively little pasta, but lots of fruits, vegetables, whole grains, fish and olive oil. So, if you were envisioning pizzas and plates of spaghetti with meatballs, think again.

There are very few head-to-head comparisons, but I would rate it as slightly healthier than a lacto-ovo vegetarian diet. It may not be quite as healthy as a vegan diet, but it is likely to be easier for most people to follow.

Now, let's turn our attention to two more healthy diets with somewhat specialized applications – the DASH and MIND diets.

The DASH and MIND Diets

DASH stands for Dietary Approaches to Stop Hypertension. As the name suggests, the DASH diet was designed to prevent high blood pressure, and reduce blood pressure if it is elevated. The DASH diet emphasizes fruits, vegetables and whole grains. Protein is supplied by low-fat dairy, fish, poultry, and nuts. Red meat, sweets, and sugary drinks are limited. You can think of it as an American version of the Mediterranean diet.

However, it is more than that. The Mediterranean diet represents how people traditionally ate in the Mediterranean regions of Spain, Italy and Greece. In contrast, the DASH diet was designed by experts based on the best available evidence as to how various foods affect blood pressure. DASH meal plans contain foods that are low in total fat, saturated fat, and cholesterol. The diet also contains foods that are high in fiber, potassium, calcium, and magnesium and low in sodium.

The DASH diet is a success story. It does exactly what it was designed to do. As one recent review[90] concluded: "Since the creation of DASH 20 years ago, numerous trials have demonstrated that it consistently lowers blood pressure across a diverse range of patients with hypertension and prehypertension." Another study[91] concluded that it was as effective as drug therapy for treating mild hypertension. Today the DASH diet is part of the "Evidence-Based Nutrition Practice Guideline for the Management of Hypertension in Adults"[92], and is recommended for the treatment of hypertension by every major medical organization.

Because the DASH diet was designed to reduce blood pressure, almost all the research has focused on that area. There is some evidence that it also reduces inflammation, heart disease risk, diabetes risk, and cognitive decline. It is likely to be as healthy overall as the Mediterranean diet, but outside of hypertension, the evidence is inconclusive at this point.

The MIND diet is the brainchild of Dr. Martha Clare Morris, a nutritional epidemiologist at Rush University Medical Center. She started with the Mediterranean and DASH diets because both of those diets have been shown to reduce the risk of dementia. Then she researched the literature for studies linking specific foods and nutrients to improving cognition and/or preventing dementia.

In short, she combined the brain-healthy features of the Mediterranean and DASH diets and further modified them based on the best scientific data available. She emphasized some components of those two diets and minimized others. She also modified the number of servings of some foods, based on the best available evidence.

- The MIND diet is a whole food, plant-based diet.
- It includes 10 "brain-healthy" food groups: green leafy vegetables, other vegetables, nuts, berries, beans, whole grains, fish, poultry, olive oil, and wine (in moderation; too much alcohol kills brain cells).
- It limits red and processed meats, butter and margarine, cheese, pastries and sweets, and fried and fast foods.
- It neither recommends nor discourages low-fat dairy foods and fruit other than berries. Dr. Morris notes that while those are healthy foods, they have no proven benefit for preventing cognitive decline.

Dr. Morris has published a study[93] comparing the effectiveness of the MIND, DASH, and Mediterranean diets at slowing cognitive decline and reducing Alzheimer's risk. She enrolled 923 participants, ages 59 to 98 years (average age = 81) from retirement communities and senior public housing units in the Chicago area. All participants were free of Alzheimer's disease when the study began. At the end of 4.5 years:

1) Strict adherence to all 3 diets significantly decreased the risk of developing Alzheimer's disease. The decreased risk was:
    - 53% for the MIND diet.
    - 54% for the Mediterranean diet.
    - 39% for the DASH diet.

2) With moderate adherence to each of the diets, the MIND diet performed slightly better than the other two diets:

    - Moderate adherence to the MIND diet decreased Alzheimer's risk by 35%.
    - Moderate adherence to the Mediterranean and DASH diets had no significant effect on Alzheimer's risk.

Obviously, all 3 diets reduced the risk of developing Alzheimer's, but the MIND diet appears to offer superior protection when adherence to each of the diets was only marginal, as it often is.

In summary, all 3 diets (Mediterranean, DASH, and MIND) are healthy diets. The Mediterranean diet reduces the risk of multiple diseases. The DASH diet is best known for reducing hypertension, and the MIND diet is best known for reducing Alzheimer's risk. They are easier to follow than vegetarian diets because they are more flexible and contain more familiar foods. That is, of course, both a blessing and a curse. The blessing is that they are easier to stick with long term. The curse is that it is tempting to add in unhealthy foods. These are all whole food, largely plant-based diets. Once you start adding in sodas, pastries, fatty foods, junk, and convenience foods, you lose all the health benefits of these diets.

We have looked at the healthy, low-fat diets (vegan and other forms of vegetarianism) and the diets with moderate amounts of healthy fats and healthy carbohydrates (Mediterranean, DASH and MIND). Before we turn our attention to the low-carb diets, let's look at one more study showing just how incredibly important fruits and vegetables are for health and longevity.

The Power Of Fruits And Vegetables

Your mom told you to eat your vegetables. It seems like health experts are constantly telling us to eat more fruits and vegetables. Yet I think many of us still don't realize just how important they are for our health. Let me share a recent study that makes the importance of fruits and vegetables crystal clear. But first, let's once again pretend this was a fad diet. The marketing hype would probably look like this:

"What if you could reduce your risk of:

- Heart Disease (primarily heart attack) by 24%?
- Stroke by 33%?
- Cancer by 14%?
- Premature death by 31% (That would add approximately 3.4 years of disease-free years to your lifespan)?

Would you like to know the secret?"

The secret, of course, is a diet rich in fruits and vegetables – probably a lot more fruits and vegetables than you are currently eating. You may be saying, "That's not news. I've heard that before." Yes, there have probably been hundreds of clinical studies looking at the benefits of diets rich in fruits and vegetables. There have also been several meta-analyses that have combined the data from many individual studies to improve the statistical power of their conclusions.

However, this study[94] is unique:

- It is the largest and most comprehensive meta-analysis looking at the benefits of fruit and vegetable consumption ever undertaken.
    - It analyzed 142 published clinical studies with over 2.1 million subjects from around the globe.

  - There were 43,000 cases of heart disease, 47,000 cases of stroke, 112,000 cases of cancer, and 94,000 deaths in these studies.
- It had enough statistical power to determine even minor effects of fruit and vegetable intake.
- It is the first meta-analysis with enough data to accurately determine the optimal intake of fruits and vegetables.

What Did The Study Show?

For most of the health outcomes examined in this study, the optimal intake of fruits and vegetables was 10 servings a day. When they compared people who were consuming 10 servings a day to people who were consuming less than one serving a day:

- Heart disease was reduced by 28%.
- Stroke was reduced by 33%.
- Premature death was decreased by 31%.
- The fruits and vegetables most strongly associated with this benefit were apples, pears, citrus fruit, green leafy vegetables, and cruciferous vegetables.

For cancer, the optimal intake of fruits and vegetables was 6 servings a day. When they compared people who were consuming 6 servings a day to people who were consuming less than one serving a day:

- Cancer was reduced by 14%.
- The fruits and vegetables most strongly associated with reduced cancer risk were green vegetables such as green

beans, yellow vegetables such as peppers and carrots, and cruciferous vegetables.

The authors speculated that the relatively small reduction in cancer risk they observed may have been because they were looking at total cancer cases rather than looking at individual cancers. Previous studies have suggested that fruits and vegetables reduce the risk of some cancers much more than others.

Finally, the authors estimated that:

- 5.6 million premature deaths/year worldwide could be prevented if people consumed 6 servings of fruits and vegetables a day, and...
- 7.8 million premature deaths/year worldwide could be prevented if people consumed 10 servings of fruits and vegetables a day.

What Does This Mean For You?

When the USDA rolled out the "Food Guide Pyramid" in 1992, they recommended 2-4 servings of fruit and 3-5 servings of vegetables a day. They tried educating the American public for almost a decade to no avail. Only 3% of Americans even came close to that recommendation. In 2011 they threw in the towel and introduced "My Plate," which recommended 5 servings (2 fruits and 3 vegetables). This is also the current recommendation of the WHO and England.

"How well are we doing with this recommendation?" you might ask. The answer is "not very well." The **bad news** is the CDC estimates that less than 13% of Americans eat 2 servings of fruit and 2-3 servings of vegetables a day. An average American eats one serving of fruit a day and less than 2 servings of vegetables a day. Clearly, we have a long way to go.

The **good news** is every added serving of fruits and vegetables is beneficial. The authors of the study estimate that for every increase of 2.5 servings a day:

- Heart disease would be reduced by 8%
- Stroke would be reduced by 13%
- Cancer would be reduced by 3%
- Premature death would be reduced by 10%

If we were to increase our intake of fruits and vegetables to even 6 servings a day:

- Heart disease would be reduced by 16%
- Stroke would be reduced by 22%
- Cancer would be reduced by 13%.
- Premature death would be reduced by 27%

Now that we fully understand the health benefits of fruits, vegetables, and plant-based diets, it is time to turn our attention to the ever-popular low-carb diets. I won't discuss the Atkins diet here. In part, that is because it has been debunked by so many health professionals over the years that it has lost much of its popularity. However, the major reason is, in contrast to the diets I have just discussed, there is not a shred of evidence that it is healthy long term. When a diet has been around for 45 years and no long-term studies have been published showing it reduces the prevalence of any disease, it deserves to be cast into the dustbin of history. Its only positive attribute is more rapid initial weight loss compared to traditional low-fat diets, but that advantage largely disappears a year or two later.

Instead, I will focus on two low-carb diets that are currently popular, the Paleo and keto diets. After that, I will answer the question, "Are any low-carb diets healthy?"

Is The Paleo Diet Healthy?

It seems like everyone you talk to is following the Paleo diet or knows someone who is following the Paleo diet. It is the latest version of the low-carb diet fad. If you have been around for a few years, like me, you have seen lots of fad diets come and go. They are immensely popular for a few years. Then people discover their weight loss was temporary or they aren't any healthier, and the diet slowly fades into obscurity. Is the Paleo diet one of those fad diets that will fade into obscurity, or is it a healthy diet that will stand the test of time?

Unicorns and the Paleo Diet

I titled this section "Unicorns and the Paleo Diet" because both are myths. In fact, the Paleo diet is based on several myths.

Myth #1: **Our ancestors all had the same diet.** What we currently know as the Paleo diet is based on the diets of a few primitive hunter-gatherer societies that still exist in some regions of the world. However, when you look at the data more carefully, you discover that the diet of primitive societies varies with their local ecosystems.

The "Paleo diet" is typical of ecosystems in which game is plentiful and fruits and vegetables are less abundant or are seasonal. In ecosystems where fruits and vegetables are abundant, primitive societies tend to be more gatherers than hunters. They eat more fruits and vegetables and less meat. The assumption that starchy foods were absent in the Paleolithic diet is also a myth. For some primitive societies, starchy fruits or starchy roots are a big part of their diet. In short, our Paleolithic ancestors probably ate whatever nature provided.

Myth #2: Our genetic makeup is hardwired around the "Paleolithic diet." In fact, humans are very adaptable. We are designed to thrive in a wide variety of ecosystems. It is this adaptability that has allowed us to expand to every nook and cranny of the world.

For example, the enzymes needed to digest grains are all inducible, which means the body can turn them on when needed. Our Paleolithic ancestors may not have eaten much grain, but we can very quickly adapt to the introduction of grains into our diet.

Myth #3: Our Paleolithic ancestors were healthier than modern man. It many respects, the Paleolithic diet is healthy, as I will discuss below. However, we need to remember that our Paleolithic ancestors rarely lived past 30 or 40. They simply did not live long enough to experience degenerative diseases like heart disease and cancer. We have no idea whether a diet that served our Paleolithic ancestors well will keep us healthy into our 70s, 80s and beyond.

Myth #4: The "health" of our Paleolithic ancestors was based on diet alone. Our Paleolithic ancestors differed from us in many other ways. They were more active. They were hunters and gatherers. They had no desk jobs, no computers, no TVs. They got more sleep. They went to bed when it got dark and got up with the sun.

However, just because the Paleo diet is based on mythology does not mean that it isn't healthy. Let's look at the pros and cons of the Paleo diet.

The Pros Of The Paleo Diet

There are lots of things to like about the Paleo diet. For example:

- It eliminates sodas, fast foods, processed foods, sugar and salt. Any diet that does that is a vast improvement over the typical American diet.

- It emphasizes fresh fruits and vegetables, another big improvement over the typical American diet.
- It has a healthier profile of fats than the other low-carb diets. It favors grass-fed beef, wild-caught fish, and free-range chicken, so it has less saturated fat and more omega-3s. It also emphasizes healthy oils such as olive, walnut, avocado, and flaxseed. In this regard, it is clearly healthier than the other low-carb diets. It does include coconut oil, which is a concern. As I pointed out previously, there is no convincing evidence at present that coconut oil is healthy.
- Like most other restrictive diets that eliminate processed foods, it can give short-term weight loss, although long-term weight loss is less certain.
- It emphasizes the use of unrefined or extra virgin oils rather than refined oils. That is a plus for most oils because the unrefined oils are more likely to contain antioxidants and beneficial phytonutrients. It is, however, a concern for coconut oil because the unrefined coconut oil is more likely to contain cancer-causing aflatoxins.

The Cons Of The Paleo Diet

There are, however, some concerns about the Paleo diet. Other experts have commented on the cost and difficulty in following the diet, especially if you eat out a lot, so I won't comment on those aspects here. I will stick with nutritional concerns with the Paleo diet. The Paleo diet eliminates cereal grains, legumes, and dairy. I am always concerned with the nutritional adequacy of diets that eliminate whole food groups. For example:

- Dairy is a major source of calcium and vitamin D in the American diet. Eliminating dairy has the potential to increase the risk of osteoporosis.

- A recent Australian study[95] found that women on the Paleo diet had low intakes of calcium, magnesium, iodine, thiamin, riboflavin, and folate. A Swedish study[96] looking only at iodine status reported that postmenopausal women on the Paleo diet for two years became iodine deficient.
- Most Americans are already not getting enough of these nutrients in their diet. We can scarcely afford to eliminate foods that are good sources of these nutrients.
- It is possible to carefully design a Paleo diet so these nutrients are provided by other foods, but most people don't carefully design their daily diet.
- Whole grains, legumes and dairy are important sources of magnesium. Magnesium deficiency has the potential to increase the risk of heart disease, among other things.

I find it amusing that the Paleo diet purposely eliminates some of the most significant nutritional advances of the last generation. For example, the addition of vitamin D to dairy products has virtually eliminated rickets. The addition of iodine to salt virtually eliminated goiter. However, because our Paleolithic ancestors didn't eat dairy or iodized salt, they aren't part of the diet. The Paleo diet needlessly increases the risk of both iodine and vitamin D deficiency.

- The Paleo diet recommends increasing protein intake to 19-35% of calories. Because legumes have been eliminated, the increased protein intake is coming almost entirely from animal protein, primarily red meat and fish. As I discussed previously, a heavy reliance on red meat in any diet is a concern because red meat has been classified as a probable carcinogen. Grass-fed beef only reduces heart disease risk, not the risk of cancer. Moreover, grass-fed beef is not always available, especially if you eat out frequently. If you are not eating grass-fed beef, you will be taking in more saturated fats and the healthier fat profile of the Paleo diet will disappear.

- The Paleo diet has been influenced by the recent hype about health benefits of coconut oil. Coconut oil is just one of several oils that are recommended. However, if you look on the internet today, coconut oil is featured in almost every Paleo diet recipe. Until we have definitive evidence whether or not coconut oil is healthy, I would emphasize the other oils recommended for the Paleo diet, and use coconut oil sparingly.
- My biggest concern is that there are no studies showing the Paleo diet is healthy long term. In contrast, there are long-term studies showing that vegan, lacto-ovo vegetarian, semi-vegetarian, Mediterranean, and DASH diets decrease the risk of heart disease, diabetes, some cancers and Alzheimer's.

Summary

In summary, there is a lot to like about the Paleo diet. It is healthier than the typical American diet, and it is healthier than most of the low-carb diets. I have concerns about the nutritional adequacy of any diet that eliminates whole food groups, and I have concerns about the heavy emphasis on red meat. There is also no evidence that the Paleo diet is healthy long term.

Since the restrictions of the Paleo diet are based on mythology rather than science, my recommendation would be to loosen the restrictions on whole grains, legumes and low-fat dairy and rely less on red meat as a protein source. I would also decrease the emphasis on coconut oil, and replace it with oils we know are healthy, like olive, walnut, avocado, and flaxseed oils. If you made those adjustments, the diet would more closely resemble the Mediterranean and DASH diets, which we know are healthy long term.

Is The Keto Diet Safe?

The ketogenic or keto diet has been around for a while. It has been used to control epilepsy in children since the 1920s. Nobody is quite sure why it helps control epilepsy, but it does. Once a mainstay of therapy, it is now primarily used as an adjunct to anti-epileptic drugs.

However, recently the keto diet has gone mainstream. It's no longer just for epilepsy. It has become the latest diet fad. If you believe the claims:

- Hunger and food cravings will disappear. The pounds will melt away effortlessly and rapidly.
- You will feel great. You'll have greater mental focus and increased energy.
- Physical endurance will increase. You'll become superhuman.
- Type 2 diabetes will disappear.
- Your blood sugar, cholesterol, and triglyceride levels will improve, reducing your risk of developing diabetes and heart disease.

What's not to like? This sounds like the perfect diet. But, are these claims true? More importantly, is this diet safe?

What Is Ketosis?

Ketosis is a natural metabolic adaptation to starvation. To better understand that statement let me start with a little of what I'll call metabolism 101.

The Fed State: Here's what happens to the carbohydrates, protein and fat in our meal during the first hour or two after we have eaten.

- The carbohydrates are converted to blood sugar (glucose), which is utilized in three ways:
    - Most tissues use glucose as their primary energy source in the fed state.
    - Excess glucose is stored as glycogen in muscle and liver.
    - Glycogen stores are limited, so much of the excess glucose is stored as fat.
- A few tissues such as heart muscle use fat as an energy source in the fed state. However, most of the fat is stored in our adipose tissue.
- Protein is also used in three ways:
    - Some of it is used to replace and repair the protein components in muscle and other tissues.
    - In conjunction with exercise, protein can be used to increase muscle mass.
    - Excess protein is converted to fat and stored.

The Fasting State: Between meals:

- Most tissues switch to fats as their primary energy source. Fat stores are utilized to fuel the cells that can use fat.
- Brain, red blood cells, and a few other tissues still rely solely on glucose as their energy source.
- Liver glycogen stores are broken down to keep blood glucose levels constant and provide energy for these tissues. (Muscle glycogen stores are reserved for high-intensity exercise.)
- As liver glycogen stores are depleted, the body starts breaking down protein and converting it to glucose.

Starvation – The Problem: If the fasting state were to continue for more than a few days, we enter what is called starvation. At this point we have a serious problem. Fat stores and carbohydrate stores (liver glycogen) exist for the sole purpose of providing fuel during the fasting state. Protein, however, is unique. There are no separate protein stores in the body. All protein in our body is serving essential functions.

To make matters worse, our brain is metabolically very active. It consumes glucose at an alarming rate. Thus, large amounts of glucose are needed, even in the fasting state. If protein continued to be converted to glucose at the same rate as during an overnight fast, our essential protein reserves would rapidly be depleted. Irreversible damage to heart muscle and other essential organs would occur. We would be dead in a few weeks.

Ketosis – The Solution: Fortunately, at this point a miraculous adaptation occurs. Our bodies start to convert some of the fat to ***ketones***.

- All tissues that use fat as an energy source during fasting can also use ketones as an energy source, sometimes with greater efficiency.
- Over a period of several days, the brain adapts to ketones as its primary energy source. This greatly reduces the depletion of cellular protein needed to supply blood glucose to feed the brain.
- However, red blood cells and a few other cells still require glucose as an energy source. Essential protein reserves are still being depleted, but at a far slower pace.
- With these adaptations, humans can survive months without food if necessary.

There are a few other adaptations that make sense if we think about the dilemma of going long periods without food.

Our appetite decreases, which makes it easier to endure the absence of food. In addition, our metabolic rate decreases, which helps preserve both protein and fat stores.

What Is The Keto Diet?

Proponents of the keto diet advocate achieving a permanent state of ***ketosis*** without starving yourself. That is achievable because the real trigger for ketosis is low blood sugar, not starvation. The starting point for the ketogenic diet is low-carb, high-fat diets like Atkins. However, keto diets go beyond traditional low-carb, high-fat diets. They restrict carbohydrates even further to <10% of calories so that a permanent state of ketosis can be achieved. Basically, the keto diet:

- Eliminates grains and sugars.
- Eliminates most fruits.
- Eliminates starchy vegetables (root vegetables, corn, legumes like peas and beans, starchy vegetables like squash and yams).
- Reduces protein intake. That's because dietary protein can be converted to glucose when blood glucose levels are low.

You are left with a highly restrictive diet that allows unlimited amounts of fats, mostly saturated, some vegetables, and moderate amounts of meats, eggs, and cheeses.

The Keto Diet Is Not For Wimps

#1: You have to be committed. As noted above, this is a highly restrictive diet. You will have great difficulty following it when you eat out or are invited to a friend's house for dinner. You will also have to give up many of your favorite foods.

#2: The transition is rough. Physiological adaptation to the keto diet will take anywhere from a couple of days to a week or two. During that time, you will have to endure some of the following:

- Headaches, confusion and "brain fog"
- Fatigue
- Hunger
- Lightheadedness and shakiness
- Leg cramps
- Constipation
- Bad breath
- Heart palpitations

#3: There are no "cheat days." On most diets, you can have occasional "cheat days" or sneak in some of your favorite foods from time to time. The ketogenic diet is different. A single "cheat day" is enough to take you out of ketosis. If you want to resume the keto diet, you will need to go through the transition period once again.

Is The Keto Diet Effective?

With this background in mind, let's evaluate the claims made by proponents of the keto diet. I'll rate them on the "Pinocchio Scale." "Zero Pinocchios" means they are mostly true. "One Pinocchio" means they are half true. "Two Pinocchios" means they are mostly false.

Zero Pinocchios (Mostly True Claims):

- **Reduced hunger.** This is part of the starvation response.

- **Improved mental focus and increased energy.** In part, this is simply in contrast to the "brain fog" and fatigue of the transition phase. However, you have also eliminated all foods that can cause blood sugar swings from your diet. Blood sugar swings can affect both mental focus and energy levels.
- **Rapid weight loss.** If we focus on short term weight loss, this is true because:
    - A lot of the initial weight loss is water. Glycogen stores retain water. As glycogen stores are depleted, the water is lost along with them.
    - Most people inadvertently reduce their caloric intake on a highly restrictive diet like this. For example, fats are often consumed along with carbohydrate-rich foods (butter with toast, sour cream with potatoes, cream cheese with bagels). While it is easy to say that unlimited consumption of healthy fats is allowed, most people reduce their consumption of fats in the absence of their carbohydrate-rich companions.
    - Note: Proponents of the keto diet will tell you that the weight loss associated with the keto diet is because you are burning fat stores. You will only burn fat stores when dietary fat intake is not sufficient to meet your energy needs. In other words, you burn your fat stores when "calories in" are less than "calories out" – just as with any other diet.
- **Reversal of type 2 diabetes**. Because carbohydrates are restricted in this diet, blood sugar and insulin levels will be low. If you are on medications, those will need to be adjusted by your physician.

One Pinocchio (Half-True Claims):

- **Lower LDL cholesterol and inflammation**. The jury is out on this one. Some studies show an improvement on the keto diet. Other studies show them getting worse.
- **Increased physical endurance.** This is only true for low-intensity endurance exercise. It is not true for any exercise or event that requires spurts of high-intensity exercise. That's because:
    - o The muscle fibers used for low intensity endurance exercise can utilize ketones with high efficiency. That means you can run for miles as long as you don't care how fast you get there.
    - o The muscle fibers used for high-intensity, short-duration exercise cannot adapt to use of ketones because they lack sufficient mitochondria. They require glycogen stores, which are depleted on a keto diet. Even in endurance events like marathons most people want to sprint to the finish line. They won't be able to do that if they are on a keto diet.

Two Pinocchios (Mostly False Claims):

- **Calories just disappear when we excrete ketones in our urine:** Maximum ketone excretion only amounts to 100 calories a day.
- **Long-term weight loss.** Some long-term success has been claimed in a highly controlled clinical setting. However, most studies show:
    - o People regain some or most of the weight after 6 months to a year.

  - After 1 or 2 years, there is no difference in weight loss between high-fat/low-carb diets and low-fat/high-carb diets.
- That's because:
  - Most people cannot stick to restrictive diets long term, and this diet is very restrictive.
  - Once you go off this diet, even for a short time, your glycogen stores will be replenished, and the water weight will return along with the glycogen.
  - The reduction in metabolic rate and the reduction in muscle mass associated with the keto diet make it difficult to keep the weight off long term.
- **It is a healthy diet.**
  - This is a healthy diet only from the point of view that it eliminates most fast foods and processed foods.
  - However, any diet that eliminates 2 and a half food groups (grains, fruits, and starchy vegetables) and limits protein is setting you up for long-term nutritional deficiencies. It is possible to cover some of those deficiencies with supplementation, but supplements can never provide all the nutrients found in real food.

Is The Keto Diet Safe?

For most people the keto diet is likely to be safe for short periods, maybe even a few months. However, we need to remember that ketosis was designed as a short-term solution to starvation, not as a permanent metabolic state. I have grave concerns if the diet is continued long term.

- I have already mentioned the likelihood this diet will create nutritional deficiencies. Long term, those deficiencies could have severe health consequences.
- Proponents of the diet recommend that protein intake be limited so that "optimal" ketosis can be achieved. If the dieter does that, it will result in a gradual depletion of essential cellular protein reserves. Long term, that has the potential to weaken heart muscle, compromise the immune system, and damage essential organs.
- Ketones can damage the kidneys. In the short term, damage is likely to be minimal as long as plenty of water is consumed. However, long-term ketosis could be a significant concern for your kidneys. I have seen proponents of the keto diet shrug this off as a concern only if protein intake is excessive. They are missing the point. The problem is the ketones, not the protein.
- Long-term ketosis has the potential to cause osteoporosis. That is because the so-called "ketones" are actually organic acids except for the small amount of acetone that gives your breath a fruity smell. Organic acids must be neutralized to keep our body pH in the normal range. There are multiple mechanisms for neutralizing organic acids. One of those mechanisms involves dissolving bone and releasing calcium carbonate into the bloodstream. This slow dissolution of bone will continue for as long as someone is in ketosis.
- Proponents of the keto diet shrug this off by saying that you never get into ***ketoacidosis*** on their diet. Again, they are missing the point. Ketoacidosis simply means that the production of organic acids has become so great that the body's mechanisms for neutralizing those acids are overwhelmed. Ketoacidosis occurs in uncontrolled diabetes and can be deadly. The problem I am referring

to is the slow dissolution of bone during long-term ketosis, not a short-term crisis like ketoacidosis.

Summary

If you are considering the keto diet for weight loss, my recommendations would be to consider other equally effective, but less demanding, weight loss programs. Look for programs that help you preserve muscle mass and teach you healthy eating habits that can be sustained for a lifetime. If you do decide to follow the keto diet, only use it for a short period of time to jump-start your weight loss. Then switch to a diet program that has been clinically proven to improve your health long term, like the ones I discussed earlier.

If you are looking for a healthy diet, I would recommend one of the diets I discussed earlier. There are no studies showing the keto diet is safe long term and reasons to suspect it is unhealthy. Your health is too valuable to risk on an untested diet program.

Are Any Low-Carb Diets Healthy?

At this point you are probably wondering whether there is any evidence that low-carb diets are healthy. The answer is: Yes, there is evidence that some low-carb diets are healthy... but, not for the reasons low-carb enthusiasts give...and, not the diets they promote. Let me elaborate.

Why Are The Arguments Of Low-Carb Enthusiasts Misleading?

Most proponents of low-carb diets claim they are healthy based on improvements in blood parameters, usually things like lower triglycerides, higher HDL, lower blood glucose and insulin levels, and lower blood pressure. They sometimes claim lower LDL levels and lower levels of inflammation.

However, clinical studies are inconsistent for the effects of low-carb diets on LDL and inflammation. They then go on to extrapolate from these data to the claim their diet will reduce the risk of heart disease, diabetes, and other diseases. These extrapolations are misleading for three reasons:

#1: Most of these comparisons are with the standard American diet. As I have said previously, almost anything is better than the standard American diet.

#2: Most of these studies are short term. The comparisons are generally made during the weight loss phase of these diets or at a time when the dieters have achieved significant weight loss. That is significant because weight loss improves all those parameters. If the comparisons had been made during the maintenance phase or after most of the weight had been regained (as it usually is), the results might have been completely different.

#3: These blood parameters are imperfect indicators of disease risk. I find it particularly amusing that low-carb proponents downplay the risk of saturated fats by saying that LDL and HDL cholesterol are imperfect indicators of disease risk and then use the same indicators to predict their diet will lower the risk of heart disease.

The only accurate way to determine the effect of a diet on disease risk is to conduct long-term studies that measure the health outcomes of the diet. Those studies have been done, but they don't support popular low-carb diets like Atkins, Paleo, or Keto.

Which Low-Carb Diets Are Healthy?

There are, in fact, several long-term studies showing that low-carb diets are healthy, but only if you ditch the animal protein and animal fats, and replace them with vegetable protein and vegetable oils.

For example, a 20-year study[97] of 82,802 women in the Nurses' Health Study found that women who ate a low-carbohydrate diet that was high in vegetable protein and oils had 30% lower risk of developing heart disease compared to women who ate a high-carbohydrate, low-fat diet. In contrast, the women who consumed a low-carbohydrate diet that was high in animal protein and fat fared no better than women consuming a high-carbohydrate, low-fat diet.

A follow-up study[98] with the same group of women compared the effect of the same diets over a period of 20 years on the risk of developing type 2 diabetes. The results were very similar. Women consuming a low-carbohydrate diet high in vegetable protein and oils had an 18% decreased risk of developing diabetes. Once again, the women consuming a low-carbohydrate diet high in animal protein and fats had just as high a risk of developing diabetes as women consuming the high-carbohydrate, low-fat diet.

This may have been because women consuming a low-carbohydrate diet that was high in animal protein and fat gained just as much weight over 20 years as women consuming a high-carbohydrate, low-fat diet. In contrast, women who consumed the low-carbohydrate diet that was high in vegetable protein and oils gained much less weight. At the end of the 20-year study[97], they weighed significantly less than the women in the other two groups. This is not surprising, since we already know that vegetarians weigh less than their meat-eating friends.

However, it does run counter to what the low-carb diet promoters have been telling you. They claim their diets help you lose weight. You do lose weight more rapidly on a typical low-carb diet, but at the end of a year or two you end up weighing just as much as if you had followed a low-fat diet[99]. These data suggest that by the end of 20 years you will have gained significant weight compared to someone following a more plant-based diet[97]. It appears that the only low-carb diet likely to give you permanent weight loss is a low-carb vegetarian diet.

This is reinforced by another study[100] showing that consumption of junk foods (potato chips and fries), sodas, processed meats, red meats, butter, sweets and desserts, and refined grains was associated with weight gain over a 4-year period. In contrast, consumption of vegetables, fruits, nuts, whole grains, and yogurt was associated with weight loss.

Finally, it's not just women. A 20-year study[101] of 40,475 men found that men consuming a low-carbohydrate diet high in animal protein and fat had a 37% increased risk of developing type 2 diabetes. In contrast, men consuming a low-carbohydrate diet high in vegetable protein and oils had a 34% decreased risk of developing type 2 diabetes.

Other Healthy Low-Carb Diets

I have previously shared evidence that a Mediterranean diet reduces the risk of developing type 2 diabetes. Several recent studies have shown that a low-carbohydrate version of the Mediterranean diet is preferable for managing people who already have diabetes. For example, one recent study[102] put people who had just developed type 2 diabetes on either the low-carbohydrate Mediterranean diet or the low-fat, calorie-restricted diet usually recommended for overweight patients with diabetes. At the end of 4 years, only 44% of the patients on the low-carbohydrate Mediterranean diet required drug treatment compared to 70% in the low-fat group.

Another entry into the low-carb diet category is the eco-Atkins diet. It is a low-carbohydrate vegan diet (I find it amusing to label a diet "Atkins" when it has no meat and no saturated fat). One recent study[103] suggests it is more effective than the Atkins diet at reducing blood lipid levels and reducing blood pressure.

Summary

Let's summarize what we've learned so far. Vegan, low-fat vegan, low-carb vegan, vegetarian, and primarily plant-based diets like the Mediterranean, DASH, and MIND diets are all healthy diets. Long-term studies show they decrease your risk of developing heart disease, diabetes, cancer, and other diseases. Long-term studies also show that plant-based low-carb diets are healthier than meat-based low-carb diets. There are no long-term studies on meat-based low-carb diets and cancer risk, but we already know that red meat is a probable carcinogen and plant-based diets decrease your risk of several cancers. In short, there is no long-term evidence that the low-carb, meat-based diets decrease your risk of any disease and some evidence that they may increase your risk of disease.

Anti-Inflammation Diets

If you have arthritis, colitis, bursitis or any of the other "itis" diseases, you already know that inflammation is the enemy. Chronic, low level inflammation is also a contributing factor to heart disease, cancer, and many other diseases. Clearly, inflammation is a bad actor. It's something we want to avoid.

Obesity and diabetes are two of the biggest contributors to inflammation, but does diet also play a role? With all the anti-inflammation diets circulating on the internet, you would certainly think so. How good is the evidence that certain foods influence inflammation, and what does an anti-inflammatory diet look like?

The Science Behind Anti-Inflammatory Diets

Let me start by saying that the science behind anti-inflammatory diets is nowhere near as strong as it is for the effect of primarily plant-based diets on heart disease and diabetes. The studies on anti-inflammatory diets are mostly small, short duration studies. However, the biggest problem is that there is no standard way of measuring inflammation. There are multiple markers of inflammation and they do not change together. That means that in every study some markers of inflammation are altered, while others are not. There is no consistent pattern from one study to another. In spite of these methodological difficulties, the studies generally point in the same direction. Let's start with the strongest evidence and work our way down to the weakest evidence.

Omega-3 fats are anti-inflammatory[104-105]. The evidence is strongest for the long chain omega-3s found in fish and fish oil, but the shorter chain omega-3s found in foods like walnuts, flaxseeds, chia seeds and flaxseed oil, soybean oil, and canola oil also appear to be anti-inflammatory.

Inflammation is directly correlated with glycemic index[106]. This has a couple of important implications. The most straightforward is that refined carbohydrates and sugars (sodas, pastries, and desserts), which have a high glycemic index, increase inflammation. In contrast, complex carbohydrates (whole grains, most fruits and vegetables) decrease inflammation. No surprise there. The second implication is that it is the glycemic index, not the sugar, that is driving the inflammatory response. That means we need to look more closely at foods than at sugars. Sodas, pastries and desserts are likely to cause inflammation, but sugar-containing foods with a low glycemic index are unlikely to be inflammatory.

Fruits and vegetables decrease inflammation. This has been shown in multiple studies. At this point most of the research is centered on identifying the nutrients and phytonutrients from fruits and vegetables that are responsible for the reduction in inflammation. I suspect they are hoping to design an anti-inflammatory supplement and make lots of money. I'll stick with the fresh fruits and vegetables.

Saturated fats are inflammatory. At face value, the data on saturated fats appear to be contradictory. Some studies say that saturated fats increase inflammation, while others say they do not. However, similar to our earlier discussion on saturated fats and heart disease, the outcome of the study depends on what the saturated fats are replaced with. When the saturated fats are compared to a diet high in refined carbohydrates and sugar (the standard American diet), they do not appear to affect inflammation. However, when saturated fats are compared to omega-3 polyunsaturated fats[107] or monounsaturated fats[108], most studies show that the saturated fats increase inflammation compared to healthier fats. Clearly, saturated fats are not the best fat choice if you wish to keep inflammation in check.

I would be remiss if I did not address the claims by the low-carb diet proponents that saturated fats do not increase inflammation in the context of a low-carb diet. I just need to remind you of two things we have discussed previously:

1) The comparisons in those studies are generally with people consuming a diet high in simple carbohydrates and sugars.

2) Those studies have mostly been done in the short term, when the participants are losing weight. Weight loss decreases inflammation, so the reduction in inflammation on the low-carb diet could be coming from the weight loss alone.

The one study[77] I have found that compares a low-carb diet (the Atkins diet) with a good diet (the Ornish diet, which is a low-fat, lacto-ovo vegetarian diet) during weight maintenance found that the low-carb diet resulted in greater inflammation than the healthy low-fat diet.

Red meat is probably pro-inflammatory. Most, but not all, studies suggest that red meat consumption is associated with increased inflammation. If it is proinflammatory, the inflammation is most likely associated with its saturated fat, its heme iron content, or the advanced glycation end products formed during cooking.

What Does An Anti-Inflammatory Diet Look Like?

Anti-inflammatory diets have become so mainstream that they now appear on many reputable health organization websites such as WebMD, the Mayo Clinic, and the Cleveland Clinic. Each have slightly different features, but there is a tremendous amount of agreement.

Foods an anti-inflammatory diet includes: In a nutshell, an anti-inflammatory diet includes fruits and vegetables, whole grains, plant-based proteins (like beans and nuts), fatty fish, and fresh herbs and spices. Specifically, your diet should emphasize:

- **Colorful fruits and vegetables**. Not only do they help fight inflammation, but they are a great source of antioxidants and other nutrients important for your health.
- **Whole grains**. They have a low glycemic index. They are also a good source of fiber, and fiber helps flush inflammatory toxins out of the body.
- **Beans and other legumes**. They should be your primary source of protein. They are high in fiber and contain antioxidants and other anti-inflammatory nutrients.
- **Nuts, olive oil, and avocados**. They are good sources of healthy monounsaturated fats, which fight inflammation.
- **Fatty** fish. Salmon, tuna, and sardines are all great sources of long chain omega-3 fatty acids, which are incorporated into our cell membranes. Those long chain omega-3s in cell membranes are, in turn, used to create

compounds that are powerful inflammation fighters. Walnuts, flaxseeds, and chia seeds are good sources of short chain omega-3s. The efficiency of their conversion to long chain omega-3s that can be incorporated into cell membranes is only around 2-5%. If they fight inflammation, it is probably because they replace some of the saturated fats and omega-6 fats you might otherwise be eating.

- **Herbs and spices**. They add antioxidants and other phytonutrients that fight inflammation.

Foods an anti-inflammatory diet excludes: In a nutshell, an anti-inflammatory diet should exclude highly processed, overly greasy, or super sweet foods, especially sodas and other sweet drinks. Specifically, your diet should exclude:

- **Refined carbohydrates, sodas and sugary foods**. They have a high glycemic index, which is associated with inflammation. They can also lead to weight gain and high blood sugar, both of which cause inflammation.
- **Foods high in saturated fats**. This includes fatty and processed meats, butter, and high fat dairy products.
- **Foods high in trans fats**. This includes margarine, coffee creamers, and any processed food containing partly hydrogenated vegetable oils. Trans fats are very pro-inflammatory.
- **French fries, fried chicken, and other fried foods**. They used to be fried in saturated fat and/or trans fat. Nowadays, they are generally fried in omega-6 vegetable oils. A little omega-6 in the diet is OK, but Americans get too much omega-6 fatty acids in our diet. Most studies show that a high ratio of omega-6 to omega-3 fatty acids is pro-inflammatory.

- **Foods you are allergic or sensitive to**. Eating any food that you are sensitive to can cause inflammation. This comes up most often with respect to gluten and dairy because so many people are sensitive to one or both. However, if you are not sensitive to them, there is no reason to exclude whole grain gluten-containing foods or low-fat dairy foods from your diet.

What Does This Mean For You?

In case you didn't notice, the recommendations for an anti-inflammatory diet closely match the other healthy diets we have discussed. It should come as no surprise then that both the Mediterranean[109,110] and DASH[111] diets are anti-inflammatory. Vegan and vegetarian diets also appear to be anti-inflammatory as well. The anti-inflammatory nature of these diets undoubtedly contributes to their association with a lower risk of heart disease, diabetes, and cancer.

As for the low-carb diets, the jury is out. There are no long-term studies to support the claims of low-carb proponents that their diets reduce inflammation. The few long-term studies that are available suggest that low-carb diets are only likely to be anti-inflammatory if vegetable proteins and oils replace the animal proteins and fats that are currently recommended.

What does this mean for you if you have severe arthritis or other inflammatory diseases? An anti-inflammatory diet is unlikely to "cure" your symptoms by itself. However, it should definitely be a companion to everything else you are doing to reduce inflammation.

What Do Blue Zones Tell Us About Diet?

Are you confused yet? I have done my best to cut through the confusion of the dueling diets based on the best possible science, but there is still a fundamental problem in interpreting the studies behind each of these diets. The long-term studies underpinning the plant-based diets are mostly association studies. They compare groups of people consuming two different diets and ask what health outcomes are associated with the diets. As I discussed earlier, association studies can be misleading.

In contrast, the popular low-carb diets are based on short-term studies. The proponents of these diets are extrapolating from those short-term studies 20 or 30 years into the future and predicting possible health outcomes, which is uncertain at best.

What if you took the opposite approach? What if you started with centenarians? What if you asked people living healthy, active lives well into their 100s what they ate and how they lived? Someone has done just that. His name is Dan Buettner. He identified five regions of the world, which he called "Blue Zones," where an unusually high percentage of people live into their 100s. He then asked the centenarians in each region about their diet and lifestyle. The results of this remarkable study were published in a book called "The Blue Zones."

How Was The Blue Zone Study Done?

Dan Buettner is not a scientist. He is a journalist, and his initial "Blue Zone" expeditions were sponsored by National Geographic. However, to his credit he collaborated with the top scientists in the fields of demographics, social anthropology and statistics. In short, he did things right.

The demographers helped him locate the Blue Zones and pored over the birth and death records, so they could prove beyond a shadow of a doubt these were regions where an extraordinary percentage of people lived to 100 and beyond. The social anthropologists helped him design the questionnaires and interview the centenarians. The statisticians helped him analyze the data.

The Blue Zones were very diverse. They consisted of:

- A mountainous municipality on the Island of Sardinia off the coast of Italy.
- Rural villages on the Island of Okinawa.
- The Seventh-day Adventist community in Loma Linda, California.
- Some remote villages in Costa Rica.
- A small island called Ikaria off the coast of Greece.

Many of these locations are remote, but the Seventh-day Adventist community lives in the heavily populated Los Angeles basin. In his book, Dan Buettner describes getting off the freeway and driving past all the usual fast food restaurants on his way to interview the Seventh-day Adventist centenarians, who obviously never ate at those restaurants.

The people in each of these regions followed a lifestyle that was dramatically different from people in surrounding communities. In the case of the Seventh-day Adventists, their lifestyle was based on their religious teachings. People in the other regions were simply following traditions passed down over many generations.

It is fascinating to read about each of these Blue Zone communities. There were some significant differences in the foods they ate and the way they lived their lives. However, Dan Buettner and his scientific collaborators were not interested in the differences. They were interested in the similarities.

The similarities were striking. More importantly, they tell us a lot about the kind of diet and lifestyle that is associated with health and longevity. This isn't hypothetical health and longevity based on some short-term clinical studies. This is real life health and longevity based on people who have actually lived it.

What Do Blue Zones Tell Us About Longevity?

Here are the nine common characteristics of every Blue Zone studied. I call them "the secrets of the centenarians":

#1: They engage in moderate intensity exercise every day. None of them run marathons or engage in high-intensity workouts in the gym. Some are shepherds. Others tend their farms. The Seventh-day Adventists take nature walks. Exercise isn't planned. It is part of their daily life.

#2: They stop eating before they are full. As a child, I remember a TV ad in which the actor would say "I can't believe I ate the whole thing" before plopping two Alka Seltzers into a glass of water. The long-living people in Blue Zones don't do that. They stop eating when they are no longer hungry, not when they are full. Okinawans call it *hara hachi bu*, which roughly translates into stopping when their stomachs are 80% full. That simple practice cuts calories by 20% and dramatically reduces the incidence of obesity.

#3: They eat a mostly plant-based diet. They eat mostly fruits, vegetables and whole grains. Nuts also play an important role in their diet. Beans are the major protein source. They avoid processed foods and seldom eat meat. Strict Seventh-day Adventists avoid meat entirely. The other Blue Zone populations ate meat primarily on special occasions. When they did eat meat, it was often pork or lamb. Based on the data from these Blue Zone populations, Dan Buettner recommends eating meat no more than twice a week, with each serving being the size of a deck of cards.

#4: They have a libation with their meals. For the Sardinians, it was red wine. For the Okinawans, it was sake. The key is moderation. No more than a glass or two. If you don't drink, that's fine too.

#5: They have a purpose in their lives. They have a reason to live. It can be service to others. It can be a hobby. It can be a quest for learning something new. Whatever it is, they have something to look forward to every day.

#6: They set aside time for relaxation. They have a time set aside each day to relax with friends or family and de-stress. This improves their mental outlook and reduces their risk of disease.

#7: They participate in a spiritual community. The religions were different in each Blue Zone, but they all belonged to strong religious communities. As Dan Buettner put it: "The simple act of worship is one of those subtly powerful habits that seems to improve your chances of having more good years."

#8: They put family first. They build their lives around their families, and when they become old their families take care of them.

#9: They surround themselves with communities that share their values. These social networks provide support, encouragement, and happiness.

As you read through the 9 things that these Blue Zone communities have in common, your first reaction may be one of dismay. In today's world, it is exceedingly difficult to achieve all 9 elements of a centenarian lifestyle. Just be comforted with the thought that the more of these 9 elements you can incorporate into your personal "Blue Zone," the healthier you will be and the longer you will live.

What Do Blue Zones Tell Us About Diet?

If you have been trying to figure out what kind of diet is best for you, the biggest take-home lesson from "The Blue Zones" is that you can forget all the absolutes you have heard from the proponents of various diet plans. For example:

- All the Blue Zone communities included whole grains, legumes, and starchy vegetables as part of their diet. **You don't have follow a low-carb diet to live to 100.**
- While all the Blue Zone communities ate a plant-based diet, most included some meat in their diet. **You don't have to go meatless to live to 100.**
- Some of the Blue Zone communities ate pork and lamb as their main meat. **If you eat meats sparingly as part of a mostly plant-based diet, you can eat red meat and still live to 100.**
- Only two of the five Blue Zones were in the Mediterranean region. **You don't have to follow a Mediterranean diet to live to 100.**

In short, the proponents of today's popular diet plans remind me of the fable of the 6 blind men grabbing different parts of an elephant and trying to describe the elephant. Each is describing part of the elephant, but none of them know what the whole elephant is like. When you see the entire elephant, it looks a lot different.

Summing Up The Diets

Let's summarize the pros and cons of the diets I have just discussed. It is, of course, not possible to cover all the dueling diets in a single book. However, the other popular diets are similar to one or more of the diets I have discussed. Hopefully I have given you enough information to make informed choices among these diets and the dozens of new diets that come along each year.

Plant-Based Low-Fat Diets

The Vegan Diet: This is a whole food, plant-based diet. It uses plant proteins instead of meat and plant substitutes for dairy and eggs.

Pros:

- Whole food, plant-based diet.
- Associated with lower blood pressure, blood sugar, cholesterol, triglycerides, and inflammation.
- Good for weight loss. Also, good for keeping the weight off. Vegans weigh less than their meat-eating counterparts.
- Long-term clinical studies suggest that it significantly reduces the risk of major diseases like heart disease, cancer, and diabetes. People on this diet live healthier, longer.
- A very low-fat version of this diet excludes all vegetable oils and appears to actually reverse atherosclerosis (clogging of the arteries).

Cons:

- Likely to be deficient in vitamin B12, vitamin D, and long chain omega-3 fats. Proper planning is required to assure adequate calcium and protein intake.
- Restrictive.
- Long-term adherence is relatively low, but some people are sufficiently motivated by their improved health to stick with this diet for a lifetime.

The Dean Ornish Diet. This is a very low-fat version of a lacto-ovo vegetarian diet that eliminates all oils, even vegetable oil.

Pros:

- Whole food, primarily plant-based diet.
- All the advantages of the vegan diet, plus even stronger evidence that it reverses atherosclerosis.

Cons:

- Very restrictive.
- Long-term adherence is low.

Vegetarian Diets: The term vegetarian encompasses a wide range of diets, including vegan, lacto-ovo vegetarian (dairy and eggs in addition to plant foods), pesco-vegetarian (fish in addition to plant foods), and semi-vegetarian (some meat in addition to plant foods).

Pros:

- Whole food, primarily plant-based diets.
- Good for weight loss. Also, good for keeping the weight off. Vegetarians weigh less than their meat-eating counterparts.
- All the advantages of the vegan diet. The pesco-vegetarian diet appears to be slightly more effective than the vegan diet at lowering colon cancer risk. The other versions of vegetarianism appear to be slightly less effective than the vegan diet at lowering risk of heart disease, diabetes, and cancer, but they are all very healthy diets long term.

- Less restrictive than the vegan diet so they are somewhat easier for people to follow.

Cons:

- Long-term adherence is still relatively low.

Healthy Fat, Healthy Carb Diets

The Mediterranean Diet. This diet emphasizes fresh fruits and vegetables, whole grains, fish, nuts, seeds, legumes and olive oil. It includes cheese, poultry and eggs in moderation.

Pros:

- Whole food diet.
- Clinical studies show long-term adherence to the Mediterranean diet is associated with a decreased risk of heart disease, certain kinds of cancer, diabetes, Parkinson's, and Alzheimer's disease.
- Relatively easy to follow.

Cons:

- Not designed specifically for weight loss. You will need to watch portion sizes and track calories if you want to lose weight on this diet.

The DASH Diet. This diet was specifically designed to help reduce the risk of hypertension and stroke. It is similar to the Mediterranean diet except that it restricts sodium and includes a wider range of lean meats and low-fat dairy products. It does not specifically include olive oil.

Pros:

- Whole food diet.
- Clinically proven to lower blood pressure as effectively as some blood pressure medications.
- Relatively easy to follow. Includes foods familiar to Americans.

Cons:

- Not designed specifically for weight loss. You will need to watch portion sizes and track calories if you want to lose weight on this diet.

Meat-Based Low-Carb Diets

The Atkins Diet. The Atkins diet is the granddaddy of the low-fat diets. It is a very low-carbohydrate diet that restricts sugars, grains, high carbohydrate fruits and vegetables. The allure of the diet is that it includes as much fatty meats and saturated fats as you want.

Pros:

- The Atkins diet is associated with several short-term benefits including weight loss, improved blood sugar control, and reduced cholesterol, triglycerides and blood pressure.

Cons:

- There are no studies evaluating the long-term benefits and risks of the Atkins diet. Any diet that has been around for 45 years and still has no long-term studies showing it is healthy deserves to be relegated to the dustbin.

- Weight loss at the end of one or two years is no better than for the low-fat diets.
- The high intake of saturated fat has the potential to increase the risk of heart disease and cancer.
- It is a very restrictive diet. Long-term adherence to this diet is poor. I come across lots of people who tell me they lose weight on this diet. Few have managed to stick with the diet and keep the weight off.

The Paleo Diet. The Paleo diet eliminates grains, sugars, refined oils, dairy, legumes, and starchy fruits and vegetables. Most of the protein comes from meats, but beef must be grass-fed. This reduces, but does not eliminate, saturated fat and gives a modest increase in omega-3 polyunsaturated fat. However, it does not turn red meats into health foods.

Pros:

- Whole food diet.
- The Paleo diet is associated with several short-term benefits including weight loss, improved blood sugar control, and reduced cholesterol, triglycerides and blood pressure.

Cons:

- There are no studies evaluating the long-term benefits and risks of the Paleo diet. Despite the hype, we have no idea whether it is a healthy diet.
- It eliminates two food groups, which is likely to lead to nutritional deficiencies long term.

- The high intake of red meat has the potential to increase the risk of cancer.
- It is a very restrictive diet, which means that long-term adherence is likely to be low.

The Keto Diet. The keto diet is even more restrictive than the Atkins diet. It restricts carbohydrates even further to <10% of calories so that a permanent state of ketosis can be achieved. Basically, the ketogenic diet eliminates grains and sugars, most fruits, starchy vegetables (squash, root vegetables, corn, legumes like peas and beans) and reduces protein intake. That's because dietary protein will be converted to glucose when blood glucose levels are low. You are left with a highly restrictive diet that allows unlimited amounts of fats and some vegetables and moderate amounts of red meat, eggs, and cheeses.

Pros:

- Whole food diet.
- The keto diet is associated with several short-term benefits including weight loss, improved blood sugar control, and reduced triglycerides and blood pressure.

Cons:

- There are no studies evaluating the long-term benefits and risks of the keto diet. Despite the hype, we have no idea whether it is a healthy diet.
- It eliminates multiple food groups, which is likely to lead to nutritional deficiencies long term.
- The high intake of saturated fats and the focus on red meat has the potential to increase the risk of heart disease and cancer.

- Long-term ketosis has the potential to cause kidney disease and osteoporosis.
- It is a very restrictive diet, which means that long-term adherence is likely to be low.

5

Eat, Drink, And Be Healthy

We have covered a lot of information together. Hopefully, I have been able to bust some food myths for you. Hopefully, I have also put the conflicting messages you have been hearing about nutrition and health on a sounder scientific footing. However, at this point you are probably suffering from information overload. It is time to summarize everything we have talked about into some simple take-home messages.

Before I do that, however, let me add some disclaimers. As I said at the beginning of this book, I am focusing only on diet and supplementation. Both of those are important, but they are only part of a holistic approach to our health. I fully acknowledge that weight control, exercise, stress reduction, adequate hydration, and adequate sleep are also vitally important.

Secondly, none of the advice I give is meant to come between you and your doctor. If you are healthy, I recommend an annual checkup. If you have an existing medical condition, your doctor may recommend more frequent visits. In today's health care environment, most doctors do not have time to discuss diet and lifestyle changes. They barely have time to diagnose the problem and prescribe a medication. However, that does not mean that most doctors are against diet and lifestyle changes. They know that every medication comes with side effects. They know that if you follow a healthy diet and lifestyle, they may not need to prescribe a medication, or they may be able to use a lower dose.

Doctors simply need to know you will work with them. What doctors fear most is that you will go on a "health kick" and stop seeing them. For example, let's say your doctor has told you that you need to lower your cholesterol, blood sugar, or blood pressure. You start eating better and working out. You drop a few pounds. You feel great. You may think: "Why do I need to go back to the doctor? I'm doing great." That would be an incredibly bad idea. In fact, if you don't go back for a check-up, neither you nor your doctor will know if you have been successful. That could be catastrophic!

It is good to have a conversation with your doctor and let them know that you will be co-responsible for your health. I had that conversation with my doctor years ago. Nowadays if he finds a problem, he says: "I could prescribe a medication, but here's what you can do about it." He is comfortable saying that because he knows I will do my best to make the changes he recommends and that I will be back in to see him to make sure the changes solved the problem.

Finally, if you happen to have one of the few doctors who doesn't believe that diet and lifestyle changes make a difference and just wants to prescribe medications, I have some simple advice. Find a new doctor.

Now, let's look at a few take-home lessons from this section.

#1: Avoid The Poisons. Of course, I am talking about sodas (both sugar-sweetened and diet), refined carbohydrates and sugary foods (white bread, pastries, desserts), junk foods, fast foods and convenience foods. Virtually every diet plan on the planet eliminates those foods. I have heard of "The Steak Lovers Diet," which I don't recommend, but I have never heard of a "Fast Food Lovers Diet." Nobody would think of recommending such a diet.

I use the term "poisons" advisedly. None of these foods are literally poison, but they will pack on the pounds and increase your risk of multiple diseases. However, many of you have probably grown up eating these foods. They have become "comfort" foods that are difficult to give up. Perhaps it would be better for you to think of these foods as poisons. That just might make it easier for you to follow through on the kind of dietary changes that will help you control your weight and improve your health.

#2: Ignore the Food Myths: Here is a quick review of my "Top 10 Food Myths."

1) **Chocolate**: Sorry. Eating chocolate isn't going to help you lose weight.
2) **Sugar:**
    - Sugar is sugar. There are no sugar villains, and there are no sugar heroes.
    - When it comes to the bad effect of sugars, the foods we eat are more important than the amount of sugar. Apples will always be healthier than sodas.
    - In the case of prepared foods, look for a low glycemic index rather than the amount of sugar.
3) **Diet Sodas**: Sorry. There is no good evidence that diet sodas help you lose weight and increasing evidence they may be harmful to your health. Avoid diet sodas.

4) **Saturated Fat**: The evidence is conclusive. Saturated fat from animal sources increases your risk of heart disease – even if you are following a low-carb diet. Avoid saturated fats as much as possible.

5) **Coconut oil**: There is no good evidence that coconut oil is bad for you, but there is also no good evidence that it is good for you. Use coconut oil sparingly.

6) **Protein:**

   - The warning that Americans are getting too much protein primarily applies to middle-aged couch potatoes. It would be more accurate to say that most Americans are getting too much of the wrong kind of protein (animal protein instead of vegetable protein).

   - At the other extreme, vegetarians should focus on beans, legumes, and complimentary foods as a protein source. Saying you can get all the protein you need from broccoli is incredibly bad advice, especially for seniors who need extra protein to prevent sarcopenia (age-related loss of muscle mass).

7) **Red Meat.** Sorry. There is increasing evidence that red meat consumption increases your risk of heart disease and cancer. This appears to be true even in the context of a low-carb diet. Eat red meat sparingly.

8) **Organic**: Organic foods are a better choice, but the "Certified Organic" label is no guarantee of purity.

9) **GMO**: It is better to choose non-GMO for whole foods and for proteins. Other ingredients (sugars, oils, etc.) are chemically and biologically indistinguishable from GMO and non-GMO sources. "Certified non-GMO" is also not a guarantee of purity.

10) **Label Reading**: It is a good idea to read labels, so you can avoid the truly dreadful ingredients (Artificial

sweeteners, flavors, colors, and preservatives). However, you need to aware that most internet warnings about other ingredients simply aren't true.

#3: Primarily Plant-Based Diets Are Healthier: There are variations in the specific proven health benefits for individual diets, but that statement is generally true for diets ranging from vegan to Mediterranean and DASH diets. It even appears to be true for low-carb diets. Long-term clinical studies suggest that low-carb diets which rely on vegetable protein and oils are healthier than low-carb diets which rely on animal proteins and fats.

What Is The Perfect Diet For You?

Now let's turn to the question of utmost importance to you – which diet is best for you. That, of course, depends on your goals, so I have organized this section based on possible health goals.

Weight loss: If we are talking about initial, rapid weight loss, the extremes are your best choice. Low-fat vegan and low-carb diets both are effective at helping you lose weight quickly.

- In part, that is because they exclude some of your favorite food combinations. For example, a vegan diet excludes sour cream. A low-carb diet excludes the baked potato. A vegan diet excludes the cream cheese. A low-carb diet excludes the bagel. I could go on, but I think you get the point. You eat fewer calories without thinking about it because you don't immediately replace the foods you eliminated with another food of equal calories. Eventually, most people either find alternative foods they like or go back to their old diet, and the weight comes back.

- There are practical reasons as well. With vegan diets, the lower caloric density of vegan foods makes a big contribution to weight loss. With low-carb diets, water loss makes a large contribution to the initial weight loss. Of course, that is temporary. As soon as you add back carbohydrates, you regain all the water weight you lost with the low-carb diet.

The Mediterranean and DASH diets are also healthy diets for weight loss. They also include more familiar foods than the diets at the extremes, which is both a disadvantage and an advantage.

- The disadvantage is that having so many familiar foods to choose from makes it easier to overeat, so you will need to pay more attention to portion sizes and total calories.
- The advantage is that the Mediterranean and DASH diets are easier diets to stick with long term. Long-term adherence to vegan and low-carb diets is poor at best.

In considering the best weight loss diet, it is important to ask yourself whether you are learning food choices that will allow you to maintain your weight loss and be healthy for the rest of your life. Based on those criteria, I cannot recommend the meat-based low-carb diets (see below). It also eliminates many of those widely advertised diets that rely on pre-packaged meals. Unless you have unlimited funds, you are not going to be able to buy pre-packaged, low-calorie junk food for the rest of your life.

Weight Maintenance: In terms of long-term weight maintenance, vegetarian diets win hands down. Multiple studies show that long-time vegetarians weigh less, probably because the caloric density of vegetarian diets is low. Simply put, that means you have to eat a lot more food to pack on the pounds with a vegetarian diet than with other diets. When you compare the various forms of veganism, vegans weigh the least. Lacto-ovo, pesco-, and semi-vegetarians weigh slightly more, but still significantly less than people eating the standard American diet.

With the Mediterranean and DASH diets, it is less clear. If you closely follow the restricted calorie versions of those diets you find on the web, you should be able to keep your weight in check. We just don't have the long-term data to prove it.

With low-carb diets, we do have some long-term data. Those data suggest that people following a meat-based, low-carb diet gain just as much weight over a 20-year period as people consuming a low-fat diet. In contrast, people following a plant-based, low-carb diet gain significantly less weight over the same time period.

In summary, it is clear a primarily plant-based diet is best for maintaining a healthy weight. Furthermore, you have multiple healthy options to choose from. That is fortunate because you will be most successful keeping the weight off on a diet you can stick with for a lifetime. You may need to experiment a bit to find the diet best suited for you. Once you have made your choice, you will find all the meal plans and recipes you need online, and most of that information is free.

Heart Health: Once again, plant-based diets are the best choice if you wish to reduce your long-term risk of developing heart disease. Based on comparisons of vegetarian diets from the Seventh-day Adventist Studies, it appears that the vegan diet is most effective for reducing heart disease risk, followed by lacto-ovo vegetarian and semi-vegetarian, in that order.

The Mediterranean diet is also very effective at reducing heart disease risk. It has not been directly compared to a vegan diet, but its heart health benefits appear to be similar. That is likely because it is a primarily plant-based diet plus heart-healthy monounsaturated and omega-3 polyunsaturated oils.

As for low-carb diets, meat-based low-carb diets offer no benefit at reducing heart disease risk compared to a low-fat diet. In contrast, plant-based low-carb diets decrease heart disease risk by about 30%.

If you already have heart disease and wish to significantly reduce LDL cholesterol and reverse atherosclerosis, strict adherence to either the Ornish diet or a very low-fat version of the vegan diet appear to be your best choices. If you are primarily interested in reducing blood pressure, the DASH diet is the obvious choice, based on multiple clinical studies.

Diabetes: Plant-based diets also appear to be superior at reducing long-term risk of developing type 2 diabetes. Among the vegetarian diets, the vegan diet is the most effective at reducing diabetes risk, but all forms of vegetarianism significantly reduce diabetes risk compared to the standard American diet. Once again, the Mediterranean diet is also very effective at reducing the risk of developing type 2 diabetes.

There is also a recurring theme with low-carb diets. In women, meat-based low-carb diets do not reduce the risk of developing type 2 diabetes any better than low-fat diets. In men, they appear to increase the risk compared to low-fat diets. Once again, plant-based low-carb diets decreased the risk of developing diabetes compared to low-fat diets in both men and women.

If you already have diabetes, a lower carb diet may be helpful for managing blood sugar levels. I would recommend the low-carb version of the Mediterranean diet because it has been used successfully in the management of patients with type 2 diabetes. You also might wish to consider the eco-Atkins diet. Its name is misleading. It is actually a low-carb version of a vegan diet.

Cancer: Once again, plant-based diets rule. Both vegetarian and the Mediterranean diet have been shown to reduce the risk of certain kinds of cancer. Multiple studies have shown that fruit and vegetable consumption decrease cancer risk. In contrast, processed meats clearly increase cancer risk, and many studies suggest that red meat consumption may increase cancer risk as well.

Cognitive Decline and Alzheimer's: The data are fairly limited for cognitive decline and Alzheimer's. There are studies suggesting that the Mediterranean, DASH, and MIND diets reduce Alzheimer's risk. Vegetarian diets are also likely to be beneficial, but they have not been studied in this context. There are also studies suggesting that the keto diet may be beneficial for some patients with Alzheimer's. At this point, I would probably recommend the Mediterranean or MIND diets, but that may change as more research comes along.

Epilepsy: The keto diet has a long track record of helping with childhood epilepsy. There is some evidence that it may help control epilepsy symptoms in adults as well.

You Are Unique: When I started this section, I promised you that I wouldn't be one of those "diet gurus" who claims only they know the truth. They have the perfect diet, and if you just follow their diet plan you will be slim, healthy and happy. I have debunked the myths and deceptions. I have scoured the scientific literature, so that I could offer you the best options for whatever life situation you may be in. Now, it is up to you to choose the option that is the best fit for your health goals.

However, before you choose based solely on clinical study results, I want to remind you that clinical studies report average results, and none of us are average. You are unique, and you will need to find the diet plan that works best for you. Earlier I shared a study with you showing individual variability in blood sugar response. You may remember that some people had a better blood sugar response with a banana, while others had a better blood sugar response with a cookie. A recent review[112] reported that non-diabetic patients had better weight loss results on a low-fat diet, while pre-diabetic and diabetic patients lost weight more effectively on either low-carb diets or vegetarian diets. Another recent study[113] reported that our intestinal bacteria influenced which diet was most effective. I could go on, but you get the point.

Based on the available science, my recommendation would be to choose one of the plant-based diets. However, your final choice should be based on how you feel on the diet and what your blood parameters (LDL, HDL, triglycerides, blood glucose, etc.) are once you are long past the weight loss phase of the diet. My wife and I have followed essentially a semi-vegetarian diet for years. We are in perfect health, and we feel great. We have the blood parameters of teenagers. However, I did experiment with a vegan diet recently. The vegan diet gave me digestive issues and only marginally improved my blood parameters. My diet choice is clear, but your best diet choice awaits your discovery.

Change Is Hard: The perfect diet for you may be very different than your current diet. That is a good thing because you probably wish for your health to be very different than it is now. Alternatively, you may want your health trajectory to be very different than it is now. Simply put, you want to be healthy and active in your golden years rather than sick and disabled.

However, old habits die hard. Change is always difficult. Large changes are very difficult. Some people can successfully go "cold turkey" and change everything at once. Most of us aren't like that. My advice is to make the necessary changes to your diet and lifestyle gradually. My wife and I did not change our diet overnight. We made gradual changes over several years.

I remember seeing a diet book a few years ago titled something like "One Thing." Their idea was that you change one thing a week until you got to a healthy diet. Week one you might give up sodas. Week two it might be chips. You get the point. I thought that idea made a lot of sense. However, I'm not going to tell you how to change your diet. I am going to recommend that you choose the approach that works best for you.

Never Say Never: If you are telling yourself you can never eat any of your favorite foods, you are setting yourself up for failure. However, if you tell yourself you will eat your favorite foods every weekend, you are also setting yourself up for failure. Allow an occasional splurge, but be sure it is occasional. Frequency is important when you are including unhealthy foods in your diet.

For example, I grew up eating red meat. It is something I enjoy, so I allow myself an occasional splurge. However, I don't waste my splurge on a hamburger or a flank steak. I order a small filet mignon at a fine restaurant. I only order it when someone else is paying, which means it is only on very special occasions. That decreases the frequency and increases the enjoyment. I end up eating filet mignon no more than 3 or 4 times a year. When I do order it, I order a large green salad to go with it and take half of it home for the next day. That works for me. If you have favorite foods you can't bear to eliminate for a lifetime, you just need to figure out a strategy that works for you. For those favorite foods you don't need to say "never," but you don't want to say "often."

6

What Role Does Supplementation Play?

In this book I have focused on healthy foods and healthy diets. You may think that once you are making healthier food choices and following a healthier diet, supplementation isn't necessary. After all, I have shared with you all the wonderful health benefits you gain by following a healthier diet. What more is needed? My recommendation is to add a common-sense supplementation program.

To help you understand why, I have created another graphic similar to the one I used at the beginning of the book. I will just give you a brief overview here to introduce the concept of supplementation. These topics are covered in much more detail in my upcoming book, "Slaying the Supplement Myths."

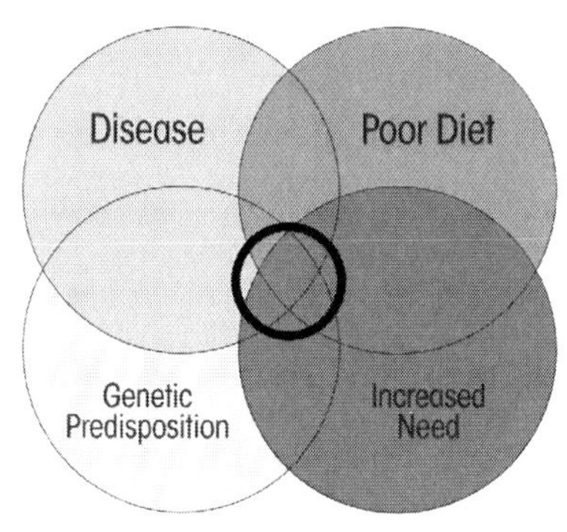

Let's start with **poor diet**. The number one reason for supplementation is to fill nutritional gaps in our diet. If you are consuming the standard American diet, junk foods, fast foods, and convenience foods have crowded out fruits, vegetables and whole grains. The USDA tells us that <10% of Americans are eating according to USDA guidelines. Consequently, the USDA tells us that most Americans are not getting sufficient amounts of calcium, magnesium, vitamin A, vitamin C, and vitamin E in our diets. More recent studies suggest that many of us are woefully deficient in vitamin D and long chain omega-3s. If you are a pregnant mom, you may not be getting enough folic acid in your diet. If you are on a weight loss program, your diet may not be nutritionally adequate simply because you are eating less food.

You may be saying to yourself: "I plan to eat a whole food diet. This doesn't apply to me." The problem is that few of us are perfect. Many people don't follow their diet plan as faithfully as they think they do. We also crave convenience, and there are food companies only too willing to sell us processed junk foods they market as perfect for whatever diet we are following. More importantly, any diet that eliminates whole food groups creates nutritional inadequacies of its own. For example, I have already discussed the nutritional inadequacies created by the vegan and Paleo diets.

Next, let's turn to **increased needs**. We have known for years that pregnancy and lactation increase nutritional requirements. Many common medications also increase our need for specific nutrients. For example, seizure medications can increase your need for vitamin D and calcium. Drugs to treat diabetes and acid reflux can increase your need for vitamin B12. Other drugs increase your need for vitamin B6, folic acid, and vitamin K. Excess alcohol consumption increase your need for thiamin, folic acid, and vitamin B6. These are just a few examples.

More worrisome is the fact that we live in an increasingly polluted world and some of those pollutants may increase our needs for certain nutrients. For example, one recent study reported that exposure to pesticides during pregnancy increases the risk of giving birth to children who will develop autism, and that supplementation with folic acid during pregnancy decreases the risk of autism[114]. (Note: One of the biggest offenders was flea and tick medicine for pets. I wonder how many women know they should not be applying flea and tick medicine on their pets while they are pregnant.) I do wish to acknowledge that this is a developing area of research. This and similar studies require confirmation. It is, however, a reminder that there may be factors beyond our control that have the potential to increase our nutritional needs.

Next, let's consider **genetic predisposition**. This is part of a fascinating new area of nutrition research called ***nutrigenomics***. Simply put, nutrigenomics is the study of how genes and nutrition interact. The best-known example of nutrigenomics is the mutations that lead to reduced activity of the enzyme methylenetetrahydrofolate reductase (MTHFR). Individuals with these mutations have an increased need for folic acid and benefit from folic acid supplementation. (Note: The popular notion that these individuals require methylfolate instead of folic acid is a myth. I discuss this in "Slaying The Supplement Myths.") There are many other examples of genetic mutations that increase our needs for certain nutrients. I discuss some of them in "Slaying The Supplement Myths."

Finally, let's consider the effect of **disease** on our nutritional needs. If you look at the popular literature, much has been written about the effect of stress on our nutritional needs. In most case, the authors are referring to psychological stress. In fact, psychological stress has relatively minor effect on our nutritional needs. Metabolic stress, on the other hand, has major effects on our nutritional needs. Metabolic stress occurs when our body is struggling to overcome disease, recover from surgery, or recover from trauma. When your body is under metabolic stress, it is important to make sure your nutritional status is optimal.

Finally, let's step back and view the whole picture. The overlapping circles are drawn that way to make a point. A poor diet doesn't necessarily mean you have to supplement. However, when a poor diet overlaps with increased need, genetic pre-disposition, or metabolic stress, supplementation is likely to be beneficial. The more overlapping circles you have, the greater the likely benefit you will derive from supplementation.

That is why I include supplementation along with diet, exercise, and weight control as part of a holistic approach to better health. I will take a deeper dive into this topic in my upcoming book, "Slaying the Supplement Myths." There are companies that have poor quality controls, companies with no evidence their supplements are either safe or effective, companies that will lie to you (they call it marketing), and companies who make supplements that are dangerous. I cover all that in a section of "Slaying the Supplement Myths" which I call "The Lies of the Charlatans." There is a tremendous amount of confusion about the benefits and risks of supplementation. I cover that in a section of "Slaying the Supplement Myths" which I call "The Myths of the Naysayers."

Glossary
(In Order Of Appearance)

Microbiome: The term microbiome refers to all the microorganisms in our body. For our purposes, microbiome refers primarily to intestinal microorganisms. Our microbiome can be influenced by diet and can, in turn, influence our health.

Metabolite: A metabolite is an intermediate or product of metabolism.

Epigenetics: For our purposes the best definition would be changes to metabolism or nutritional requirements caused by chemical modification of the DNA or proteins bound to DNA rather than by alterations of the genetic code. These chemical modifications can be influenced by diet and environment and, in some cases, are hereditable.

Paradigm: A paradigm is a framework containing the basic assumptions, ways of thinking, and methodology that are commonly accepted by members of a scientific community.

Intervention clinical study: In an intervention study, the investigators put one group of research subjects on a particular diet. Usually, they compare subjects following the diet to subjects who have not changed their diet. Then the researchers measure how the subjects' health changes.

Association clinical study (also referred to as an epidemiologic study or population study): An association study is a clinical study that compares health outcomes in populations of people. Ideally, the two population groups are matched in every way except for one variable (diet, for example). They are then compared to some health outcome. The strength of this type of study is that it allows you to study associations of diet with health outcomes in large populations over a long time. However, unexpected confounding variables (see definition) can be a problem in this type of study.

Confounding variable: A confounding variable is an extraneous variable whose presence affects the variables being studied so that the results you get do not reflect the actual relationship between the variables under investigation. As an example, suppose that there is a statistical relationship between ice cream consumption and number of drowning deaths for a given period. These two variables have a positive correlation with each other. An evaluator might attempt to explain this correlation by inferring a causal relationship between the two variables (for example, ice cream causes drowning). However, a more likely explanation is that the relationship between ice cream consumption and drowning is spurious and that a third, confounding, variable (the season) influences both variables: during the summer, warmer temperatures lead to increased ice cream consumption as well as more people swimming and thus more drowning deaths.

Carcinogen: For our purposes, a carcinogen is a substance capable of causing cancer in humans.

Carcinogenicity: For our purposes, carcinogenicity is the ability of a substance to cause cancer in humans.

Atherosclerosis: The deposition of fatty materials on the inner walls of our arteries. This restricts blood flow and increases the risk of a heart attack or stroke.

Ketones: Chemical substances that the body produces from fat when insulin levels are very low. Only one of the substances produced is a true ketone. The major substances produced are actually keto acids.

Ketosis or ketogenesis: Ketosis or ketogenesis refers to the production of ketones and keto acids from fats when insulin levels are very low. Normally, this physiological state only occurs during prolonged starvation, but it can also occur during uncontrolled diabetes or severe carbohydrate restriction.

Ketoacidosis: Ketoacidosis is a severe, systemic acidic condition that occurs when the production of keto acids overwhelms the body's ability to neutralize them. This is usually only seen in uncontrolled diabetes.

Nutrigenomics: Nutrigenomics is the study of how individual genetic makeup interacts with diet, especially the effects of this interaction on a person's health.

References

1 G.D. Wu et al, Science, 334: 105-108, 2011.

2 V. Koeth et al, Nature Medicine, doi:10.1038/nm.3145.

3 M.E. Lindholme et al, Epigenetics, 12: 1557-1569, 2014.

4 W.M. Braun et al, British Journal of Sports Medicine, 49: 1567-1578, 2015.

5 K.S. Bishop and L. R. Ferguson, Nutrients, 7: 922-947, 2015.

6 R. Do et al, PLOS Medicine, October 2011, doi/10.1371/journal.pmed.1001106.

7 A.P. Levy et al, Diabetes Care, 27: 2767, 2004.

8 S. Kreijkamp-Kaspers et al, American Journal of Clinical Nutrition, 82: 1260-1268, 2005.

[9] K. Gustafsson et al, American Journal of Clinical Nutrition, 83: 592-600, 2006.

[10] R.A. Waterland and R.L. Jirtle, Molecular and Cellular Biology, 23: 5193-5300, 2003.

[11] D.C. Dolinoy et al, Environmental Health Perspective, 114: 567-572, 2006.

[12] D.C. Dolinoy et al, PNAS, 13056-13061, 2007.

[13] E.W. Tobi et al, International Journal of Epidemiology, doi: 10.1093/ije/dyv043, 2015.

[14] Z.Y. Ong & B.S. Muhlhausler, FASEB J, 25: 2167-2179, 2011.

[15] C.O. Bondi et al, Biological Psychiatry, 75, 35-46, 2014.

[16] J. Smith et al, Journal of Clinical Endocrinology & Metabolism 94: 4275-4283, 2009.

[17] F. Guernard et al, PNAS 110: 11439-11443, 2013.

[18] D.G. MacArthur et al, Science, 335: 823-828, 2012.

[19] D. Zeevi et al, Cell, 163, 1079-1094, 2015.

[20] T.E. Strandberg et al, European Journal of Clinical Nutrition, 62: 247-253, 2008.

[21] M. Kazuhiko et al, Nutrition Research, 31: 122-130, 2011.

[22] B.A. Golomb et al, Archives of Internal Medicine, 172: 519-521, 2012.

[23] J.A. Greenberg et al, PLOS ONE, 2013, 8(8) e70271.

[24] I. Aeberli et al, American Journal of Clinical Nutrition, 94: 479, 2011.

[25] R.A. Forshee et al, American Journal of Clinical Nutrition, 89: 438-439, 2009.

26 D.P. DiMeglio et al, International Journal of Obesity, 24: 794-800, 2000.

27 M.B. Schulze et al, JAMA, 292: 927-934, 2004.

28 V.S. Malik, American Journal of Clinical Nutrition, 89: 438-439, 2009.

29 V.S Malik, Diabetes Care, 33: 2477-2483, 2010.

30 T.T. Fung et al, American Journal of Clinical Nutrition, 89: 1037-1042, 2009.

31 Q.Yang et al, JAMA Internal Medicine, 174: 516-524, 2014.

32 S.P. Fowler et al, Obesity 16: 1894-1900, 2008.

33 R. Dingra et al, Circulation, 116: 480-488, 2007.

34 M.Y. Pepino et al, Diabetes Care, 36: 2530-2535, 2013.

35 E. Green & C. Murphy, Physiology & Behavior, 107: 560-567, 2012.

36 S. Basu et al, American Journal of Public Health, 103: 2071-2077, 2013.

37 D.C. Greenwood et al, British Journal of Nutrition, 112: 725-734, 2014.

38 B. Xi et al, PloS One, 9:e93471, 2014.

39 F. Imamura et al, British Journal of Medicine, doi: 101136/bmj.h3576, 2015.

40 H. Gardener et al, Journal of General Internal Medicine, 27: 1120-1126, 2012.

41 M.P. Pase et al, Stroke, DOI: 10.1161/STROKE.AHA.116.016027.

42 M.C. Borges et al, PLOS Medicine, DOI: 10.1371/journal.pmed.1002195.

[43] R. Chowdhury et al, Annals of Internal Medicine, 160: 398-406, 2014.

[44] M.U. Jakobsen et al, American Journal of Clinical Nutrition, 89: 1425-1432, 2009.

[45] F.M. Sacks et al, Circulation. 2017;135.00-00. DOI: 10.1161/ CIR.0000000000000510.

[46] K.N. Porter Starr et al, The Journals of Gerontology, Series A, 71: 1369-1375, 2016.

[47] T.M. Longland et al, American Journal of Clinical Nutrition, 103: 738-746, 2016.

[48] A. Dougkas et al, The Journal of Nutrition, 146: 637-645, 2016.

[49] W.W. Campbell et al, Journal of Gerontology: Medical Sciences 56A: M373-M380, 2001.

[50] S. Katsanos et al, American Journal of Clinical Nutrition, 82: 1065-1073, 2005.

[51] T.B. Symons et al, American Journal of Clinical Nutrition, 86: 451-456, 2007.

[52] T.B. Symons et al, Journal of the American Dietetic Association, 109: 1582-1586, 2009.

[53] C.S. Katsanos et al, American Journal of Physiology, Endocrinology & Metabolism, 291: E381-E387, 2006.

[54] D.K. Layman et al, Journal of Nutrition, 133: 411-417, 2003.

[55] D.K. Layman et al, Journal of Nutrition, 135: 1903-1910, 2005.

[56] D.A. Lasker et al, Nutrition Metabolism, 5: 30, doi: 10.1186/1743-7075-5-30, 2008.

57 D.K. Layman et al, Journal of Nutrition, 139: 514-521, 2009.

58 E.M. Evans et al, Nutrition Metabolism, 55: doi: 10.1186/1743-7075-9-55, 2012.

59 M.C. Mojtahedi et al, The Journals of Gerontology A: Biological Sciences and Medical Sciences, 66: 1218-1225, 2011.

60 M.M. Mamerow et al, Journal of Nutrition, 144: 876-880, 2014.

61 S.M. Pasiakos *et al*, The FASEB Journal, 27: 3837-3847, 2013.

62 R. Jagr et al, Journal of the International Society of Sports Nutrition 14:20, 2017. DOI: 10.1186/s12970-017-0177-8, 2017.

63 M. Baranski et al, British Journal of Nutrition, 112: 794-811, 2014.

64 D. Ornish et al, Lancet, 336: 129-133, 1990.

65 D. Ornish et al, Journal of the American Medical Association, 280: 2001-2007, 1998.

66 H.S. Dod et al, American Journal of Cardiology, 105: 362-367, 2010.

67 C.R. Pischke et al, Journal of Cardiovascular Nursing, 25: E8-E15, 2010.

68 C.B. Esselstyn et al, Journal of Family Practice, 41: 560-568, 1995.

69 C.B. Esselstyn et al, Journal of Family Practice, 63: 356-363, 2014.

70 G.E. Fraser, Journal of Nutrition Health & Aging, 9: 53-58, 2005.

71 S. Tonstadt et al, Nutrition Metabolism & Cardiovascular Disease, 23: 292-299, 2013.

72 R.Y. Huang et al, Journal of General & Internal Medicine, 31: 109-116, 2016.

73 M.J. Orlich et al, JAMA Internal Medicine, 175: 767-776, 2015.

74 W.J. Craig, American Journal of Clinical Nutrition, 89(Supplement): 1627S-1633S, 2009.

75 M.J. Orlich and G.E. Fraser, American Journal of Clinical Nutrition, 100(Supplement 1): 353S-358S, 2014.

76 L.T. Le and J. Sabate, Nutrients, 6: 2131-2147, 2014.

77 M. Miller et al, Journal of the American Dietetic Association, 109: 713-717, 2009.

78 P.N. Singh et al, American Journal of Clinical Nutrition, 78 (Supplement 3): 526S- 532S, 2003.

79 M.J. Orlich et al, JAMA Internal Medicine, 173: 1230-1238, 2013.

80 S. Mihrshahi et al, Preventive Medicine, 97: 1-7, 2017.

81 C.M. Kastorini et al, Atherosclerosis, 248: 87-93, 2016.

82 R. Estruch et al, The New England Journal of Medicine, 368: 1279-1290, 2013.

83 K. Esposito and D. Giugliano, Diabetes/Metabolism Research and Reviews, 30 (Supplement 1): 34-40, 2014.

84 P.A. van den Brandt and M. Sculpen, International Journal of Cancer, 10: 2220-2231, 2017.

85 M. Qaqundah, Natural Medicine Journal, 9: Issue 5, 2017.

86 S. Gallus et al, European Journal of Cancer, 13: 447-452, 2004.

87 R.N. Alcalay et al, Movement Disorders, 27: 771-774, 2012.

88 N. Scarmeas et al, Annals of Neurology, 59: 912-921, 2012.

89 N. Scarmeas et al, Neurology, 69: 1084-1093, 2007.

90 D. Steinberg et al, Journal of the American Medical Association, 317: 1529-1530, 2017.

91 F.M. Sacks et al, New England Journal of Medicine, 344: 3-10, 2001.

92 S.L. Lennon et al, Journal of the Academy of Nutrition and Dietetics, 117: 1445-1458, 2017.

93 M.C. Morris et al, Alzheimer's & Dementia 11: 1007-1014, 2015.

94 D. Aune et al, International Journal of Epidemiology, 46: 1029-1056, 2017.

95 A. Genomi et al, Nutrients, 8, 314; DOI:10.3390/nu8050314, 2016.

96 S. Manousi et al, European Journal of Clinical Nutrition, DOI: 10.1038/ejcn.2017.134.

97 T.L. Halton et al, New England Journal of Medicine, 355: 1991-2002, 2006.

98 T.L. Halton et al, American Journal of Clinical Nutrition, 87: 339-346, 2008.

99 F.M. Sacks et al, New England Journal of Medicine, 360: 859-873, 2009.

100 D. Mozaffarian et al, New England Journal of Medicine, 364: 2392-2404, 2011.

101 L. de Koning et al, American Journal of Clinical Nutrition, 93: 844-850, 2011.

[102] K. Esposito et al, Annals of Internal Medicine, 151: 306-314, 2009.

[103] D.J.A. Jenkins et al, Archives of Internal Medicine, 169: 1046-1054, 2009.

[104] I. Reinders et al, European Journal of Clinical Nutrition, 66: 736-741, 2011.

[105] B.K. Iariu et al, American Journal of Clinical Nutrition, 96: 1137-1149, 2012.

[106] L. Qi and F.B. Lu, Current Opinion in Lipidology, 18: 3-8, 2007.

[107] J.A. Paniagua et al, Atherosclerosis, 218: 443-450, 2011.

[108] B. Vessby et al, Diabetologia, 44: 312-319, 2001.

[109] L. Gallard, Nutrition in Clinical Practice, 25: 634-640, 2010.

[110] L. Schwingshael and G. Hoffmann, Nutrition Metabolism and Cardiovascular Diseases, 24: 929-939, 2014.

[111] D.E. King et al, Archives of Internal Medicine, 167: 502-506, 2007.

[112] M.F. Hjorth et al, American Journal of Clinical Nutrition, 106: 491-505, 2017.

[113] M.F. Hjorth et al, International Journal of Obesity, DOI: 10.1038/ijo.2017.220, 2017.

[114] R.J. Schmidt et al, Environmental Health Perspectives, DOI: 10.1289/EHP604, 2017.